How to . . .

get the most from your
COLES NOTES

Key Point
Basic concepts in point form.

Close Up
Additional hints, notes, tips or background information.

Watch Out!
Areas where problems frequently occur.

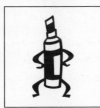

Quick Tip
Concise ideas to help you learn what you need to know.

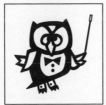

Remember This!
Essential material for mastery of the topic.

Your Guide to . . .

Yoga

25 yoga postures

Breathing & nutrition

Relaxation & meditation

COLES NOTES have been an indispensable aid to students on five continents since 1948.

COLES NOTES now offer titles on a wide range of general interest topics as well as traditional academic subject areas and individual literary works. All COLES NOTES are written by experts in their fields and reviewed for accuracy by independent authorities and the Coles Editorial Board.

COLES NOTES provide clear, concise explanations of their subject areas. Proper use of COLES NOTES will result in a broader understanding of the topic being studied. For academic subjects, COLES NOTES are an invaluable aid for study, review and exam preparation. For literary works, COLES NOTES provide interesting interpretations and evaluations which supplement the text but are not intended as a substitute for reading the text itself. Use of the NOTES will serve not only to clarify the material being studied, but should enhance the reader's enjoyment of the topic.

© Copyright 2002 and Published by
COLES PUBLISHING. A division of Prospero Books
Toronto – Canada
Printed in Canada

Cataloguing in Publication Data
Fedosoff, Janie, 1961-

Your guide to ... yoga: 25 yoga postures;
breathing & nutrition, relaxation & meditation

(Coles notes)
Written by Janie Fedosoff and Ilse Gordon
ISBN 0-7740-0601-3

1. Yoga, Ha.tha. I. Gordon, Ilse, 1941-. II. Title. III. Series.

RA781.7.F42 2000   613.7'046   C00-930292-1

Publisher: Nigel Berrisford
Editing: Paul Kropp Communications
Book design: Karen Petherick, Markham, Ontario
Layout: Christine Cullen
Illustration: Kent Monkman, Christine Cullen

Manufactured by Webcom Limited
Cover finish: Webcom's Exclusive DURACOAT

Contents

Chapter 1   **What is yoga?**   1
Classifying the yogas
The "Om" symbol
The hara center

Chapter 2   **The importance of the breath**   8
Pranayama – the yogic science of breath control
Abdominal breathing
The complete breath
Sun and moon breath

Chapter 3   **What you need to start your yoga practice**   17
A special note for menstruating women

Chapter 4   **25 yoga postures (asanas) with illustrations**   20
1. *Total Relaxation Posture*
2. *Spread Leg Stretch*
3. *Back Stretch*
4. *Cobra*
5. *Plough*
6. *Dog*
7. *Bow*
8. *Bridge*
9. *Boat*
10. *Wheelbarrow*
11. *Shoulder Stand*
12. *Spinal Twist*
13. *Laughasana*
14. *Lion*
15. *Cat*
16. *Child Posture*
17. *Thigh Stretch*
18. *Squatting Posture*

Chapter 4   *19. Mountain Pose*

                20. Classical Forward Stretch

                21. Back Bend

                22. Triangle

                23. Warrior

                24. Tree

                25. Easy Posture

Chapter 5   **Yoga programs to suit your needs**   74

                Program A: to start your day and energize
                    your mind and body

                Program B: to end your day and release tension

                Program C: for quick stress reduction

                Program D: for slimming the body

                Program E: to strengthen the back and spine

                Program F: to help release negative emotions

                Program G: for pregnant women

Chapter 6   **Nutrition for yoga and better health**   95

                Guidelines for eating before and after exercise

                Everyday diet considerations

                Traditional yoga nutrition and principles

                Vegetarianism

Chapter 7   **Affirmations**   102

Chapter 8   **Relaxation**   106

                Basic relaxation technique

                Tension / relaxation exercise

Chapter 9   **Meditation**   110

                How to meditate

                Chakras and chakra meditation

CHAPTER ONE

What is yoga?

Yoga is an ancient practice that is Indian and Hindu in origin. Around 200 BC, a sage named Patanjali created a manual of 196 aphorisms called the Yoga Sutras, which form the basis of all systems of yoga philosophy and practice. The ultimate goal of yoga for a Hindu mystic is to attain a life of total absorption in Brahman, a Sanskrit term that means the Absolute, the One or the Universal Spirit.

As a Westerner, you may not be interested in reaching the lofty spiritual goals of a Hindu yogi, but you can still practice one of the many disciplines of yoga for the simple goal of improving your physical health. For instance, regular practice of the postures that comprise the physical aspect of hatha yoga promotes a healthy body and mind. However, through the regular practice of yoga, you will achieve other benefits that are at the heart of yogic teachings – greater physical and mental health resulting from better lifestyle choices.

Yoga has evolved from relative obscurity in Western society to become a popular form of exercise for men and women of all ages. You are probably most familiar with hatha yoga. Hatha yoga is best known for the postures or asanas that comprise the physical aspect of its practice. When you think of yoga, you may picture a quiet, relaxed environment permeated with the aroma of incense and the sound of gentle music. This image is quite accurate because hatha yoga is a relaxing method of exercise that is ultimately designed to quiet the mind.

CLASSIFYING THE YOGAS

Yoga can be both an end-goal to be reached – enlightenment – and a system of disciplines and techniques practiced to reach the end-goal. There are many different yoga disciplines because there are different types of individuals who desire enlightenment. The main yogas can be identified as follows:

Jnana yoga	Union by knowledge
Bhakti yoga	Union by love and devotion
Karma yoga	Union by action and service
Mantra yoga	Union by voice and sound
Yantra yoga	Union by vision and form
Laya yoga	Union by arousal of latent psychic nerve-force
Raja yoga	Union by mental mastery
Hatha yoga	Union by bodily mastery, principally of breath

Jnana yoga is best suited to those with an intellectual temperament as it follows the path of spiritual knowledge and wisdom. To practice this form of yoga, the student makes use of conscious reasoning to penetrate the veils of ignorance and illusion that prevent him from seeing the light of pure consciousness that yogins consider the basis of life. The practitioner of Jnana yoga must develop his intellect through study and meditation to transcend his ego and find his True Self (Atman).

Bhakti yoga is based on devotion, worship and love of God. A practitioner of Bhakti yoga will focus his devotion on a wor-shipped deity like Krishna for Hindu practitioners or Jesus Christ for Christian practitioners. The disciplines of Bhakti yoga include following ancient rites, singing songs of praise or hymns and regular prayer. This form of yoga has a natural appeal to people with strong religious and spiritual temperaments.

Different cultures practice Bhakti yoga in different forms. Hindus express devotion by singing hymns of praise, dancing and repeating japa, the rhythmic repetition of mantras. According to Bhakti yoga there is no difference between Christ, Buddha, Allah or any other deity; all are believed to equally represent God. The Bhakti yogin enjoys a love of music and art as a manifestation of God and believes that focusing on a constant love of God will ultimately bring him closer to Samadhi, meaning enlightenment or self-realization.

Karma yoga may be the most difficult form of yoga for

Westerners, as it requires following a path of selfless service and action, without consideration of personal gain. There is a close connection between Bhakti yoga – the yoga of love and devotion – and Karma yoga – the yoga of selfless action.

A Karma yogin considers work a gift of God. He or she performs tasks for others without the expectations of reward or acknowledgment of any kind. (If one expects a reward, this leads to expectation and attachment, which in turn leads to suffering.) The emphasis of Karma yoga is on the action being performed with full intention, in the here and now, and in the spirit of love, care and compassion. Mother Theresa and Mahatma Ghandi are considered excellent examples of Karma yogins.

Mantra yoga may be the easiest yoga to follow. The practitioner chants or recites a mantra to activate and accelerate the creative spiritual force within and to promote harmony in all parts of her being. Mantras can be repeated vocally, either loud or soft, or thought inwardly. The aim is to empty the mind of all other thoughts and feelings. By excluding these other distractions, the practitioner will achieve absorption into the Universal Conscious Energy.

A mantra is a precise combination of words and sounds that are the embodiment of a particular form of consciousness. Mantras are a combination of sacred syllables considered to possess spiritual potency. Gurus, Holy Ones and Rishies (beings of a higher state of consciousness) have passed these down to us over the ages. Common mantras include:

Om: this is the first sound of the universe

Om Shanti Shanti Shanti: refers to peace in three aspects – physical, mental and spiritual

Hari Om: a healing mantra that calls on the preserving power of the Divine to maintain the body and mind in the highest state of health possible, for the purpose of self realization.

When repeating a mantra, the sound should come from the heart and penetrate each cell of the body.

Yantra yoga uses sight and form the way Mantra yoga uses the vibration of voice and sound. A yantra can be a picture, object or inner visualization that holds the power to influence the consciousness of the observer. In Northern India and Tibet colorful mandalas are the contemplative objects of Yogins. The symbol of the Cross may hold the same powerful influence for Christian followers in Western society.

Laya yoga is symbolically linked to the Hindu deity Shiva, the destroyer. Shiva destroys the bondage of the ego. The abode of Shiva is in the area just above the skull, outside the physical body. Shakti, a force issuing from Shiva, moves through the head in a descending direction and manifests in the bottom of the spine. This energy, stored and coiled like a serpent at the base of the spine, is referred to as Kundalini Shakti. In most people this energy is dormant. The object of Laya yoga is to reawaken the Kundalini energy and move it from the base of the spine up through the seven major chakras (whirling energy centers) to reach samadhi (enlightenment or self-realization).

Raja yoga is also referred to as the Royal Path because the person who practices this method of yoga aims to become the ruler over his own mind. This form of yoga involves mastering consciousness and stilling the mind. Other yogas have the same intent but use practices that involve other physical and spiritual aspects to help the practitioner to gain control of the mind.

To practice raja yoga you must quiet your thoughts, empty your mind and reduce internal disturbances until the surface of your mind is calm. When this state is achieved, the white light of pure consciousness can shine in with all its purity. The practitioner of this yoga becomes an observer of the thoughts that enter the mind. By being aware of this flow of thoughts, it becomes possible for the practitioner to weed out negative and destructive thoughts. These interfering thoughts are referred to as maya (illusion of the mundane world of everyday living).

Hatha yoga is the yoga of body control. Its aim is to create perfect balance within. The word *hatha* is derived from Ha representing the sun, inhalation, masculine and positive properties and Tha representing the moon, exhalation, feminine and negative properties. Through hatha practice, the practitioner will balance

4

these opposing forces and thus reaches samadhi.

Hatha yoga has three important aspects and these will be covered in this book:

Asanas To get to know one's body and become aware of it. This term refers to the postures and to the place where the postures are performed. Asanas provide the opportunity to become aware of your body.

Breathing Pranayama (prana means universal energy).

Diet A vegetarian diet is encouraged for both health and compassionate reasons.

Hatha yoga appeals to Western culture because it focuses on physical well-being, and the benefits extend naturally to promote a healthier state of mind. This includes better concentration and a more positive outlook on life.

Through the continued practice of the asanas, the body becomes stronger, more flexible and poised. This increased strength allows you to sit still comfortably, for increasing periods of time. Developing the ability to sit without fidgeting is an important component to meditation and relaxation.

The mastery of proper breathing techniques, cleansing processes to remove toxins from your body and healthy eating habits are also important to the study of hatha yoga. All these disciplines create the groundwork for following the other paths of yoga and eventually reaching the superior aim of all yoga, samadhi or enlightenment.

THE "OM" SYMBOL

Om is a sign, a symbol and a secret key. It is the deepest sound of cosmic music, a universal sound of existence. All mantras are to begin and end with this key word. Om signifies the ultimate reality of the Creator and repeating and meditating on this sacred sound will eliminate all obstacles on a person's path to the awakening of a new consciousness.

The *Mundaka Upanishad* states: *Om is the bow, the individual self is the arrow, and the spirit is the target. One should then become one with it, like the arrow that has penetrated the target.*

Om was the first sound of the universe. It is how the letters A, U and M are jointly pronounced. Each of these letters is devoid of spiritual force, but together they arouse energizing vibrations.

A   represents the earth. This is pronounced as a guttural sound.

U   represents heaven. The lips thrust forward when you make this sound.

M   represents the divine, beyond all senses. It is formed by closing the lips together, causing a resonant tone like the humming of a bee.

It is recommended that this mantra be recited every morning, evening and prior to bedtime. Through this practice, you charge your nervous system with positive vibrations that reduce stress in body and mind. When the mind is quiet and empty of thoughts, cosmic energy starts to descend and penetrate the nervous system. The benefits include hormonal regulation and regeneration of nerve cells, resulting in very deep sleep. Blood pressure is reduced and the internal organs are relaxed.

THE HARA CENTER

There are many forms and centers of subtle energy that you can learn about if you choose to extend your knowledge of yoga beyond the basics contained in this book. However, if you don't gain a basic understanding of the hara center, you will never achieve the balance that is the focus of all yoga practice. The hara center is known by many different names: the original energy center in some meditation teachings, the *tan tien* in Tai Chi, the second brain in some philosophies. This is your most important energy center, and oxygen, blood and energy are naturally drawn to this area of the body. However, if this energy center is depleted, it will immediately replenish itself by drawing energy from other organs in the body, leaving these organs depleted.

The hara center is the true center of your physical and subtle energy bodies, your true point of balance. It is located internally in the area three finger-widths below the navel and approximately 2.5 to 3.5 centimetres inside the body. You can rejuvenate this center through deep breathing, mindful relaxation, meditation and laughing.

The word *hara* comes from the Japanese and literally means belly. Hara is thought of as more than a point of balance, it is considered a state of balance. People unconsciously feel secure around someone who speaks from the belly. In North American culture, we refer to the gut and the importance of paying attention to our gut feelings.

In your everyday life it is important to focus on your hara. Pay attention to maintaining a feeling of balance. When things get too stressful or crazy, simply stop for a moment and focus your breathing into the hara center. Let the weight that you are holding in tension around your shoulders and upper body consciously drop to the feet and then focus on the midpoint of your body. Breathe deeply into the hara center for a few moments, and then return to your tasks with a more relaxed attitude. Ultimately you should learn to function from the hara at all times, to achieve true balance in your life.

Before you start practicing yoga

Prior to commencing any new form of physical activity, it is wise to consult your doctor. The regular practice of any forms of yoga can bring you great health benefits. However, your doctor can advise you of any potential risks. This is particularly important when beginning hatha yoga and the asanas described in this book.

CHAPTER TWO

The importance
of the breath

PRANAYAMA – THE YOGIC SCIENCE OF BREATH CONTROL

Prana – a Sanskrit term – is defined as life breath or vital air.
Prana is more than just air; it is the life force that permeates
everything in the universe. Pranayama is the knowledge and control
of prana by which samadhi may be achieved. Learning to breathe
properly is at the very foundation of yoga. You must practice and
master some basic breathing techniques in order to gain the true
benefits of any other yoga practice.

Humans may live for days without water, and weeks without
food, but our life would end in minutes if we were unable to breathe.
So it is interesting that Western culture puts so little emphasis on
proper breathing techniques. Most people instinctively know to take
a deep breath to relax but only use one-ninth of the lung's capacity
for normal breathing. Slow, deep breathing relaxes the limbic system,
the emotional center of the brain, and as a result your body shifts
from a fight-or-flight response to a relaxed response. By practicing
yogic breathing techniques you can learn to make every breath more
effective, help reduce overall stress and also receive a great deal of
additional health benefits.

The basics of the respiratory system

To gain a better understanding of yogic breathing techniques, it
is helpful to understand the basic physiology of how our respiratory
systems work. Your upper body, often called the trunk, is made up of
two main parts: the abdominal cavity and the thoracic cavity. The
lungs are suspended within the thoracic cavity and have no ability to
contract on their own. It is the action of the ribs, intercostal muscles

and the diaphragm that creates a vacuum, thus filling the lungs with air. The diaphragm is the thick muscle at the base of the thoracic cavity. When it contracts, it descends toward the abdominal cavity and this increases the amount of space in the chest. This increased space creates a pressure change between the lungs and the chest wall and air fills the expanded lungs to normalize the pressure. If you breathe without fully engaging the action of the diaphragm muscle, you will breathe in shallow, short breaths. When our breath is shallow it indicates that we are stressed and continuing to breathe this way causes increased stress. One of your first lessons in yoga is to learn to use the diaphragm for deeper, more effective breathing.

Humans have both automatic and conscious control of breathing. Automatic control is triggered by the brain and feedback from our lungs, muscles and the oxygen-carbon dioxide levels in our blood. This automatic control allows us to continue to breathe while sleeping or unconscious. Our conscious control is what we use for talking, singing, laughing and many other uniquely human functions. However most of us are still largely unaware of our conscious breath control. Yoga teaches you to observe and control your breath so you can enjoy its many health benefits as a result.

Good posture promotes good breathing.
When you slouch, you compress the lungs,
resulting in a loss of energy.

Our lungs contain millions of tiny air sacs called alveoli around which blood flows. When we inhale, these tiny sacs fill with oxygen and transfer it to the oxygen-depleted blood cells around these air sacs. The blood then transports this oxygen to the cells of the body along with the nourishment from any food we have eaten. Through the process of osmosis, the tissues and cells take oxygen and nourishment from the blood in exchange for their waste. Carbon dioxide in the blood is carried back to the lungs while other waste products are deposited in other waste removal organs, like the liver and kidneys. When the carbon dioxide-laden blood cells return to the sacs around the lungs, the reverse happens and carbon dioxide is absorbed into the sacs and exhaled out of lungs. This is a perfect nutrition and waste management system that most humans take for granted.

When we smoke, eat improper food and fail to exercise, this perfect system breaks down. We starve our cells of the nutrients and oxygen they require and we fail to remove all of the toxic waste from our system. When we are stressed out, we also fail to exhale completely, leaving stale air in our lungs. This also causes a buildup of toxicity in the body and results in irritability, confusion and fatigue. This increased toxicity is directly linked to many chronic illnesses. Just learning to breathe better greatly improves the efficiency of this system and your overall health.

Prana means vitality and life force, and *ayama* means control of this life force. Prana contains all the minerals the body requires for maintenance – iron, magnesium, zinc, etc. It is wise to make use of this. The morning air contains the most prana, so it is good to work on your breath early in the day.

In the interest of improving our health, there is little we can do to change the oxygen content of the air we breathe, but we can greatly improve the capacity of the lungs and thus the amount of oxygen we provide to our blood. Deep-breathing exercises are one of the most effective ways to improve the muscles of the respiratory system and the capacity of the lungs.

1. Breathe through the nose, not the mouth. Your nose filters and warms the air before it enters your lungs.
2. Practice in a well-ventilated area with an abundance of the cleanest air available.
3. Do not eat before you practice; a half-empty stomach is best.
4. Relax. Do not practice to the point of exhaustion or excess strain.
5. Don't get discouraged – keep practicing. You have been breathing the same way for most of your life, so it will take you some time to change.

Caution

If you have lung, heart, eye or ear troubles or suffer from high blood pressure, make sure you do not pause between exhalation and inhalation. As well, inhalations and exhalations should be moderate in length.

In the beginning, **do not** practice these breathing exercises for longer than three minutes at a time or you may start hyperventilating. You need to increase the capacity and strength of your lungs and diaphragm slowly.)

ABDOMINAL BREATHING

This is also referred to a diaphragmatic breathing. Using this technique you will learn to use your diaphragm more effectively to fill your lungs with air and provide your body with more oxygen. This technique is also used in the hara center breathing described in Chapter 1.

If you want to observe this technique in another person, watch someone, in particular a baby, sleeping on his back. You will see that this is the natural way we breathe when we are truly relaxed. When you start to observe your breath regularly, you should also notice how shallowly you breathe during times of stress. To counter that stress, simply stop what you are doing and do some abdominal breathing exercises. You should notice an immediate stress reduction. Once you learn to breathe into the abdomen, this can be done lying, sitting, standing or walking.

Technique

1. Lie on your back with your legs extended – see the *Savasana* or Total Relaxation Posture (asana 1). Allow the feet to fall away from each other to open up the pelvic area. Your chin is slightly down to release pressure from the neck and shoulders.

2. Place both hands flat on the area of your navel with the tips of the longest fingers touching. You are learning to move this area to affect your breathing so that each time you inhale, your fingertips separate. Each time you exhale they touch again. This will help you recognize your progress. Likewise you can rest a book on your abdomen to observe the rise and fall with each breath. Later, once you have mastered the movement of the abdomen, allow your arms to rest beside the body, with the palms facing up to open up the shoulders.

3. Relax into the floor and close your eyes so that you focus only on your breathing. Release any tension.

4. Inhale through the nostrils and feel your abdomen expanding at the same time. You may exaggerate this motion while you are learning to cultivate this technique. Breathe in a slow, steady manner to the count of four. Observe the motion of the abdomen by watching the book rise or feeling the separation of the fingertips during the inhalation.

5. Exhale to the count of four and release, allowing the stomach to become concave, emptying all of the air out of your lungs. Your exhalation should equal your inhalation. This is a deep-breathing exercise focusing on the abdomen and filling the deepest parts of the lungs with air – your shoulders and upper chest **do not** move.

6. Feel your body relaxing more and more with each exhalation.

7. Try to do this at least three to five minutes each day.

Initially you may find it very difficult to feel or see any movement in your abdomen but do not be discouraged – you have probably been breathing incorrectly for many years. As you become more skilled in abdominal breathing, try to practice in a seated or standing position and finally incorporate it into your everyday life. Driving a car, waiting in line, holding on the phone are all perfect times to practice since you will improve your skill level and reduce the stress associated with these activities at the same time.

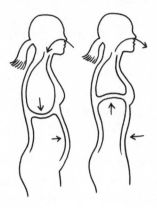

THE COMPLETE BREATH

Begin to practice this breath only after you have become comfortable with the abdominal breath. The aim of the complete breath is to fill the lungs with as much prana or vital energy as possible and to eliminate stale air from the lungs and toxins from the body. Continued practice will increase your conscious control of your breath and improve your everyday breathing.

The complete movement should find you conscious of all the working parts and muscles of your respiratory system, having first the feeling of fullness followed by the feeling of emptiness in the lungs. Your inhalation should only be carried to the point of fullness without strain and the exhalation should feel as though the lungs have been completely emptied. It is important to inhale and exhale slowly, particularly at the transition of each inhalation to exhalation and exhalation to inhalation. Do not gasp at the start of an inhalation or quickly expel a lot of air at the start of an exhalation – aim for an even flow of air in and out. First master the complete breath lying down; then sitting with your back straight; and finally standing in the Mountain Posture (asana 19) – this is the most difficult.

Technique

Think of your upper body as having three main sections – the abdomen; the intercostal area between the diaphragm and the heart; and the upper area from the heart to the collarbone. In this exercise you concentrate on progressively filling each section with an equal amount of air until your lungs are completely full, without straining to the point of discomfort. Throughout the breath visualize the intake of vital energy and clean air, and the expulsion of toxins and stale air. Or you may want to visualize a white color entering the lungs. This is the color of the energy of the lungs, representing the purity and cleanliness of prana. When exhaling, visualize a grey color emerging from the lungs, representing the stale, toxic air from deep in your lungs that you are expelling and replacing with prana.

1. Begin lying down in the Total Relaxation Posture (asana 1).
2. Close your eyes, relax and center yourself. Exhale completely.
3. Slowly inhale through the nose – this should be to a count of four. First allow the abdomen to fill, allowing it to balloon out like it does with the abdominal breath. Next let the ribs move outwards as you fill the intercostal area. Place your hands on the ribcage and feel the sideways expansion of this area. Finally fill the upper lungs beneath the shoulders. **Do not** raise your shoulders up at any time during this breath. Each of the three areas should be filled with one-third of the total breath.

You must learn the complete breath in three stages. First focus on filling only the abdominal section, to a count of four. This may take several weeks to master. Then fill only the abdominal and intercostal areas until you have mastered the next level. And finally work on filling all three sections, as described above.

4. Exhale to the count of four, reversing the order of the inhalation. Your goal is to empty the upper region, middle region and finally the abdominal region of the lungs.
5. Squeeze out as much stale air as possible by collapsing the abdomen so it becomes concave and pulling the diaphragm muscle up under the ribcage.
6. Do not practice for longer than three minutes in the beginning to prevent hyperventilating.

The length of the count for inhalation and exhalation is unique to each person. Use the four count as a guideline but only work to your capacity and experiment with what is comfortable to you. Strive to gently increase the count of the breath as your lung capacity and tone improves.

SUN AND MOON BREATH

Like all yogic practice, the overall goal of the sun and moon breath is balance. It has long been known in the ancient yoga teachings that one nostril is always dominant when we are breathing. If we are healthy then this dominance switches from one nostril to the other every two hours.

To understand this, moisten your wrist and place it close to your nose, now exhale. You should be able to feel a stronger flow of air from one nostril. You may even notice that the air from the right side is warmer. This is because the right side is associated with the sun and represents a positive force. The left side is cooler and associated with the moon or a negative force. When this balance is interrupted you can suffer various effects. When the right side dominates you may feel hot, nervous or distraught. When the left side dominates you may feel cold, tired and lethargic. The goal of the sun and moon breath is to bring your breathing back into balance.

Technique

1. Sit in a comfortable position with your back straight. This can be cross-legged, the lotus position or in a straight-back chair.
2. Your right hand is placed in front of your face with the index and middle finger resting between the eyebrows. Your ring finger and little finger rest on the fleshy part of the left nostril and your thumb rests on the fleshy part of the right nostril.
3. Close the right nostril by pressing your thumb against it. Inhale steadily through the left nostril for the count of four. Fill your lungs using the same graduated technique of the complete breath, starting with the abdomen, then the middle ribcage or intercostal area of the chest and finally the upper lungs.

4.   When you complete the inhalation, close the left nostril by pressing your ring and little fingers against it.
5.   Release the thumb from the right nostril and exhale through it to the count of four.
6.   Inhale steadily to the count of four, through the right nostril, keeping the left nostril closed.
7.   When you complete the inhalation, close the right nostril by pressing your thumb against it.
8.   Release the left nostril and exhale to the count of four.
9.   This is a complete round. In summary:

- Inhale left for four
- Exhale right for four
- Inhale right for four
- Exhale left for four

Do three rounds, breathing slowly, deeply and quietly.

CHAPTER THREE

What you need to start your yoga practice

Yoga is a relatively inexpensive activity but there are a few things you will require in order to get the most benefit from your practice.

First, you want to find a quiet, well-ventilated place in your home where you can regularly practice yoga. The area needs to be large enough for you to lie down and perform the postures without restriction or fear of bumping something fragile (including your body). You may want to make this area special by lighting a candle, playing some gentle, relaxing music and eliminating anything that reminds you of stressful situations. Think of this area as your personal sanctuary; it may not feel like it when you start yoga, but after a few months this area will have a special meaning for you. Reduce the number of sudden interruptions by unplugging the phone, ignoring the doorbell and closing the door of your special room.

Second, you may want to purchase a mat if the area is not carpeted. Specialty yoga mats are available – they provide comfort when you lie or sit on the floor and can keep you from slipping while holding a posture. It is important to be able to comfortably hold a posture without fear of losing your stance. Suddenly slipping out of a posture can lead to injury. If you prefer to wear shoes, choose ones that will provide comfort and grip or work in your bare feet if the floor is not cold.

Incense, fresh flowers, plants and pictures are just a few of the other subtle, relaxing additions to enhance your yoga space and help make it special for you.

Teachers and classes Is it necessary to have yoga teacher? To increase the quality of everyday living with yoga posturing, a book like this is almost sufficient to provide all the instruction you need. But there are advantages to joining a class, especially if you are not a disciplined person. One advantage is the importance of learning proper alignment for each posture. Sometimes you think you are in correct alignment, but you are not, and a teacher will help you improve posture. The body tries to compensate for weaknesses and imbalances wherever it can – only a teacher can help you overcome this. The benefits of having a teacher also apply to meditation.

You can usually find classes offered through local recreation centers, continuing education programs and private yoga schools. Most classes meet one to two times per week and are designated as introductory, beginner, intermediate or advanced. You will also find programs for yoga instructors – these are definitely advanced. Unlike standard credit courses, you are not graded and expected to advance to the next level. You may feel comfortable staying in a beginner's class for many sessions prior to moving into an intermediate class. You may also stay at a particular level simply because it is offered at a convenient time or because you like the instructor. Your progress is dependent on your level of fitness, flexibility and willingness to learn. Do not compete or compare your progress with that of others – this is a highly individual process.

Classes are usually offered as a series that consist of a limited number of classes per session (10 to 20) for a set price, or you may find a drop-in class where you can pay as you go. If you are not disciplined you may want the additional commitment that comes from paying for a series of classes rather than one at a time. This also gives you a chance to become familiar with the instructor and others in the class. Costs can vary widely, based on where you live and the instructor or organization that sponsors the program. A little research into what is available in your area may be required to find the program that meets your budget. But don't sacrifice quality for cost – your long-term health may depend on it.

Hatha yoga is not the only form of yoga that includes a routine of postures designed for physical fitness. You may find other forms of yoga classes advertised. Some of these can be very physically demanding and are designed for the real fitness enthusiast. Make sure any yoga program you join meets your physical ability and general interest.

You should look for a yoga instructor who is certified through a reputable organization and who has practiced yoga for many years. When you are considering an instructor, ask a lot of questions about their training and background. Find out if their style and approach to yoga, exercise and lifestyle is appropriate for your goals. For instance, if a yoga instructor is highly motivated by discipline and tough workouts, and you are looking to relax and socialize, this is probably not a good fit for you and you should look elsewhere. You may have to work with an instructor for at least one session before you can determine if you will be comfortable in the class over a long term. Fortunately yoga is a growing area of interest for many and the number of qualified instructors and programs offered are increasing every year.

A SPECIAL NOTE FOR MENSTRUATING WOMEN

It is not recommended that you practice yoga when you are menstruating. The reason for this is that many of the asanas put pressure on the abdominal area and this can increase the blood flow.

- Do not perform exercises that compress the abdomen either by extreme forward or back stretches or exercises that require a lot of abdominal strength.

- Do not do any inverted postures where the head is lower than the heart. These all act on redirecting the ajana energy upward. At this time of month, there is a concentration of ajana energy moving down and out and that is why you feel less energetic. This is a natural state for the body and should not be resisted or ignored.

- The Squatting Posture (asana 18) is excellent for relieving cramps and other menstrual disorders. Practice this posture in combination with the complete breath - observing the rhythmic flow of your inhalation and exhalation to create a state of calmness and stillness.

CHAPTER FOUR

25 yoga postures (asanas) with illustrations

"If you look after the root of the tree,
the fragrance and flowering will come by itself.
If you look after the body,
the fragrance of the mind and spirit will come of itself."

– *Author unknown*

Always use common sense when practicing the asanas described below. Never strain past your physical limits. Remember that yoga is a non-violent practice that teaches you to respect your body. Do each asana to the best of your ability; recognize and accept your limits; and enjoy the process, discipline and meditative qualities of yoga practice.

Read the complete description and directions for each posture at least twice before attempting it. Study the diagram to ensure that you understand the final position you are working toward. Each posture is explained in four phases with basic rules for each phase.

When you start practicing a posture, you can spend a little time familiarizing yourself with each phase until you are comfortable with it before moving to the next phase. In other words, become comfortable with the starting position before you try the basic posture. Once you feel good about the basic posture, work on aligning the body and holding the posture, and so on. Avoid sudden, jerky movements and always release yourself slowly.

Start

Always take three deep, relaxing breaths before beginning each move. Make sure your body is correctly aligned. You may experience some discomfort in tense muscles or problem areas during the execution of an asana. It should disappear when you release the pose and become passive. This is healthy pain. Unhealthy pain occurs when you force a stretch, or attempt an asana without using the proper technique. The pain is long lasting and easily aggravated.

Basic posture

This will give you the basic instructions for attaining the posture as shown in the diagrams.

Align and hold

To complete the posture you need to align your body position, breathe deeply and hold the posture without excessively straining the body. Use common sense when judging how far to stretch your body to perform an asana.

Release

Releasing the posture properly is very important. Always exhale deeply as you slowly release the asana. A sudden, quick release from a posture can cause injury and muscle strain.

 It is imperative to relax completely by taking three deep breaths before repeating each posture. A relaxed muscle stretches much further and more easily than a tense muscle.

General thoughts on yoga practice Yoga is about learning discipline more than anything else. The physical postures of hatha yoga teach you about discipline and concentration while bringing you in touch with your body. When you are practicing the yoga postures, observe yourself before and after each asana. Have an attitude of whole-hearted attention to each movement. Refrain from clenching your teeth, tensing your jaw or frowning. Unlike competitive sports, yoga is passive and you should have an attitude almost sacramental each time you practice. Relax and enjoy working with your body. Remember, this body is yours for life. You cannot purchase another after you have damaged this one.

1. TOTAL RELAXATION POSTURE (SAVASANA)

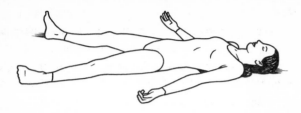

The general idea behind this posture is to lie in a state of total stillness. Remaining physically motionless for a period of time will eventually calm an agitated mind. The distractions and stresses of modern civilization make this apparently easy posture among the most difficult to master.

Benefits
✓   invigorates and refreshes both mind and body
✓   If you feel particularly fatigued after practicing a group of asanas, go into this posture for at least 10 minutes to help rejuvenate yourself.
!   If you cannot lie flat on the floor, place a support underneath your knees or neck, to make it more comfortable.

Start
Lie flat on your back on the floor with your legs stretched out but not rigid. Your feet should be slightly apart and each foot is allowed to fall outward in a relaxed manner – this opens up your pelvis. Place your palms face-up to open the shoulders. Your chin should be slightly down toward the chest to release any tension in the back of the neck.

Basic posture
1. Release yourself from all responsibilities for the next few minutes. Your conscious mind has the power to control your muscles, so you must send a message to the muscles to "let go."
2. Give all of your attention to your body. You are going to work your way from your feet to your head, consciously relaxing each part of your body. Focus first on your feet. Breathe into your feet and feel the tension begin to drain away as you slowly exhale.

Next focus on the legs, then the torso, shoulders and arms. It helps to tense each area first, then release to increase the sensation of letting go. As you progress, feel your body sinking into the floor.

3. Visualize your throat and neck relaxing. Let your lower jaw hang loose to relax it. (This is an area where you may hold a lot of tension by unconsciously clenching your teeth, while you're awake and sleeping.) Feel your mouth, eyes, forehead and finally your scalp release and relax. Feel the energy of your smile in your eyes.

Align and hold

4. As you maintain this posture, focus on your hara center – remember this is the most important energy center in the body. You will energize it through deep breathing. Use the complete breath described in Chapter 2 for this exercise. Inhale to the count of four and exhale to the count of four. Do this three times. You can rest your hands on your abdomen, as you did in the abdominal breathing exercise, with the fingertips touching. The fingertips should separate by as much as five centimetres when you inhale. This will help you focus on the expansion of the abdomen and hara center. After a few seconds, place your arms gently beside your body. Feel your spine, behind the hara center, relaxing toward the floor as you exhale.

5. After three complete breaths, resume your normal breathing rhythm and give yourself permission to enter a deep state of relaxation where rest, repair and release can take place. Do not fall asleep, you want to train the mind to remain relaxed, but aware.

Release

6. **Do not jump up** when you are finished. Your release should be slow and gentle. Start by opening the eyes and leaving them relaxed.

7. Then stretch your body, with your arms above your head and your toes pointed. Let out a big yawn.

8. Bend your knees and gently roll over to one side. Relax in this position for 10 to 15 seconds.

9. Gently push yourself up into a sitting position.

2. SPREAD LEG STRETCH (UPAVISTHA KONASANA)

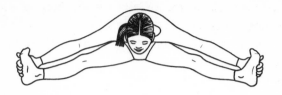

This posture is very effective for stretching the inner thigh muscles.

Benefits

✓   stretches the lower spine and hamstrings

✓   increases blood circulation in the pelvic region

✓   prevents the development of hernias

✓   relieves sciatic nerve and back pain

✓   regulates menstrual flow and stimulates the ovaries (this posture is extremely beneficial to women)

!   Proceed with caution if you suffer from fused vertebrae or hiatus hernia.

Start

1. Begin in a sitting position and spread your legs as far apart as possible. Your feet should be flexed back toward the face, arms are at your side. Straighten and elongate your spine.
2. Exhale.
3. Inhale as you raise your arms in a wide arc out from the sides of the body until they are directly overhead.
4. Stretch your arms up until you can feel the stretch in your arms and fingertips. Elongate your spine and align the body.

Basic posture

5. Exhale as you tilt your pelvis forward, making the back concave. Keep your head between your arms, continue to stretch the arms forward and elongate your spine as you lower your torso forward. Do not bounce or strain.

Align and hold

6. Based on your level of flexibility, take hold of your thighs, ankles or feet. Allow yourself to relax into this posture. Keep your knees facing the ceiling and the back of your knees pressing downward toward the floor.
7. Breathe normally and continue to draw your body closer to the floor.
8. Hold for 30 seconds.

Release

9. Release the posture and return to your original sitting position the same way you moved into it.
10. Stretch your arms above your head by raising them in a wide arc to the side of the body.
11. Inhale as you raise your arms and exhale as you slowly lower them to the resting position. Maintain a straight spine and rest.
12. Repeat three more times.

Variation

Start from a sitting position, legs spread apart, and turn your hips to the right. Align your hipbone with the center of your knee and the toe next to your big toe. Inhale as you lift your arms above your head, and elongate your spine by stretching right to the fingertips. Gently stretch over your right leg. Depending on your flexibility, take hold of your thigh, ankle or foot. Hold, breathe normally and relax into the pose. Use your hands to draw your body closer to the leg and increase the stretch in your back. Bring your chest toward the thigh instead of your head toward your knee, to keep the spine as straight as possible.

Hold for 30 seconds and release. Inhale and stretch the arms over the head; exhale and slowly return them to the resting position. Rest, keeping the spine straight, and repeat the stretch over the left leg. Repeat three more times for each leg.

3. BACK STRETCH (PASCHIMOTTANASANA)

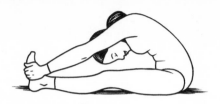

The heart of quadruped animals is located below their spine and this position keeps their heart strong and gives them great endurance. In humans, the spine is vertical and the heart is not below the spine. This causes us to feel the effects of exertion more easily and makes us more susceptible to heart disease. Yoga postures like the Back Stretch position our heart below the spine and help us develop some of the heart strength and endurance of quadrupeds.

Benefits

✓   stimulates the peristaltic movement of material through the digestive tract and prevents constipation

✓   massages the intervertebreal discs and aids in circulation of blood in this area

✓   corrects minor back disorders and stimulates the kidneys

✓   develops flexibility of the spinal column

✓   increases the amount of oxygenated blood brought into the pelvic area (the gonad glands absorb additional nutrition from this increased blood flow, which increases vitality)

!   Proceed with caution if you have fused vertebrae or hiatus hernia.

The Back Stretch is very similar to the Spread Leg Stretch.

Start

1.   Begin in a sitting position with both legs extended in front and your feet flexed back toward your face. Your legs and feet should be together and your arms are at your side.

2. Straighten and elongate your spine and exhale.
3. Inhale as you raise your arms in a wide arc out from the sides of your body, until they are directly overhead. Stretch your arms up as much as possible, until you can feel the stretch right to your fingertips. This helps to elongate the spine and correctly align the body for the posture.

Basic posture

4. Start to breathe out, tilt your pelvis forward, making the back concave. You should feel the stretch in your lower spine.
5. Keep your head between your arms, continue to stretch your arms up and forward and elongate the spine as you lower your torso toward your legs. Do not bounce or strain.

Align and hold

6. Take hold of your thighs, ankles or feet – depending on your flexibility – and relax into this posture.
7. Breathe normally, use your hands to stretch your back a little more and hold for 30 seconds.

 Maintain the extension of the legs and torso. Continue to stretch your torso forward. Press the back of your knees into the ground and keep your kneecaps and toes pointing directly up toward the ceiling.

Release

8. Release the posture and return to your original sitting position.
9. Inhale and raise your arms over your head in a wide arc out from the sides of the body. Stretch your arms up and elongate the spine.
10. Exhale as you slowly lower the arms to a resting position.
11. Rest while maintaining a straight spine, then repeat three more times.

4. COBRA (BHUJANGASANA)

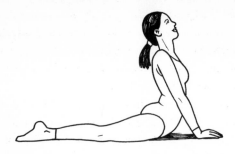

This posture is so named because it makes the practitioner resemble a cobra as it rears back to strike. The cobra is honored and revered in the East for guiding the Buddha during meditation. The muscles that are focused on include the biceps, pectoral, trapezius, latissimus dorsi and lumbar triangle.

Benefits

✓　strengthens the muscles of the back, shoulders and neck, and thus can help prevent back pain

✓　helps correct deviations of the spine and improve circulation to the intervertebral disks

✓　lowers blood pressure

✓　brings additional blood to the pelvic region, nourishing all internal organs, particularly the ovaries; helps relieve menstrual irregularities and constipation

✓　stretches the esophagus, an area of the body we rarely stretch

!　**Do not** practice the Cobra if you suffer from neck fusion, whiplash or hiatus hernia.

Start

1. Lie face down with your toes pointed backward, your feet together and your forehead touching the floor.

2. Place your palms flat on the floor directly under the shoulders (as if you were going to do push-ups). Fingertips are aligned with your shoulders; the middle fingers point straight forward. Keep your elbows as close to the body as you can.

Basic posture

3. Gently brush your forehead forward on the floor, then your nose and finally your chin.

4. Stretch your neck forward like a turtle, and stretch your entire spine forward. The goal is to create as much space between each of the spinal vertebrae as possible before you begin to raise your head, chest and trunk.

5. Inhale and keep stretching the spine forward as you slowly raise your head and chest. Use your back muscles and gently push yourself up with your arms. Feel your chest expanding as you gently bend back from the waist.

6. Stretch the top of your head away from the shoulders. Look forward and slightly up, stretching the front of the neck, and relax the spine.

Align and hold

7. Tighten your buttocks; press the pubic bone down; tighten the thigh muscles and keep the knees straight throughout the posture. Your pelvic bones stay on the floor. Maintain the stretch in your legs and arms. Express your chest. Curve your spine without putting strain on the lumbar region.

8. Breathe deeply and hold the posture for 30 seconds.

Release

9. Exhale as you release and slowly come down vertebrae by vertebrae. Your head is the last part of the body to come down.

10. When your head reaches the floor, turn it to one side and let your entire body rest on the floor while you take three deep breaths.

11. Repeat three more times.

5. PLOUGH (HALASANA)

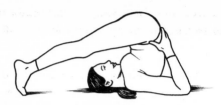

The Plough is one of the most rejuvenating of all the postures. You will be stretching your entire spine and pushing your heels away from the buttocks to enhance the stretch in your legs. This posture also provides the best stretch for the spine of any yoga posture.

Benefits

✓   stimulates the endocrine system, liver, spleen and reproductive organs

✓   helps alleviate menstrual disorders and helps muscular rheumatism

✓   prevents ossification of the vertebrae

✓   stretches arteries and veins in the legs

✓   reduces body fat

!   Do not attempt the Plough if you have severe neck problems or fused vertebrae.

Start

1.   There are two ways to start this posture. The easiest method is to start from a sitting position, inhale and roll backward to attain the basic posture. (As you progress with this posture you can start by lying on your back, arms resting beside the body with your palms facing down. Make sure your feet are together.)

2.   Take three deep, relaxing breaths.

Basic posture

3.   Inhale before you start. The impetus of your feet going over your head will force the breath out as you get into the posture.

4.   From the lying position, exhale and lift your legs up over your

head until your toes touch the floor behind your head. Keep your feet together. (If you are starting from a sitting position, your arms are resting beside you, palms down. Roll backward until your feet are behind you.) If you cannot reach the floor with your feet, just go as far as you can in comfort.

Align and hold

5. Support your back with your hands for the duration of the posture. Keep your elbows as close to the body as you can.
6. Keep your legs straight and push your heels away from the buttocks.
7. Your toes are tucked under and pointing toward your head.
8. Breathe normally and relax into the position.
9. Hold for 30 seconds.

Release

10. As with all asanas, the process of release is slow, without any jerky movements. Bend your knees until they rest beside your ears or forehead.
11. Release the arms by returning them to the start position (they will be beside the body when you are finished).
12. Bring the hips down to the floor without lifting your head, by rolling the spine on the floor, vertebrae by vertebrae.
13. When your hips touch the floor, straighten the legs upward.
14. Exhale and slowly lower your legs (with the feet together) toward the floor. Keep your lower back firmly pressed against the floor.
15. Relax by taking three deep breaths.
16. Repeat three more times. Try to consciously let go a little more each time you do this posture.

Variation

When you feel ready, you can release your hands from supporting the back and stretch them straight back in the opposite direction from the feet. Palms should be facing up.

6. DOG (ADHO MUKHA SHVANASANA)

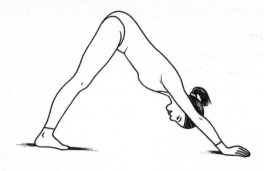

Anyone who has watched a dog stretching and playing in the park will recognize why this posture is named Dog. In Sanskrit, *adho* means downward and *mukho* means face, which is very descriptive of this posture.

Benefits

✓ strengthens, firms and tones the back, neck, abdomen, hips and legs

✓ activates the pituitary, thyroid and parathyroid glands, helps reduce body fat and brings blood to the brain cells

✓ alleviates insomnia, resting the heart and relieving tiredness

✓ especially beneficial for runners after a long, tiring race (if you are tired, hold the posture longer to help rejuvenate your energy)

! Do not practice the Dog if you have a detached retina or a tendency to suffer from dizziness. If you have high blood pressure or are menstruating, do not hold the posture. Simply follow the instructions to complete the posture and slowly release.

Start

1. Lie face-down on the floor with your feet hip-width apart and your hands underneath your shoulders.
2. Come up on your hands and knees, with your arms and thighs perpendicular to the floor and at right angles to the body. The

knees are hip-width apart and the hands are shoulder-width apart. Your middle fingers should be pointing forward. Tuck your toes under the feet.

Basic posture
3. Slowly lift the hips while straightening your arms and legs.
4. Lift the pelvis as high as you can.
5. Keep the tailbone pointing up, creating an inverted-V shape with the body.

Align and hold
6. Breathe deeply and relax into the posture.
7. Elongate your spine and neck, and stretch the head away from the shoulders.
8. Press the tailbone up (maintain equal pressure on your arms and legs). Then gently press the ribcage closer to the legs, narrowing the inverted V.
9. The heels should be pressed to the floor, toes stretched forward and the entire foot aligned facing forward. The hands are also aligned forward with the weight pressing on the heels of the hands and the thumb.
10. Distribute your weight evenly over all four points. As you breathe, the diaphragm moves up into the chest cavity and the heart rate slows down.
11. Breathe deeply and maintain this posture for at least 30 seconds.

Release
12. With a long, slow exhalation, stretch your trunk forward and lower your body gently to the floor. Your knees should touch the ground first.
13. Lie face-down, turn your head to the side and let the floor support your body weight.
14. Breathe deeply and repeat after you take three deep breaths.
15. Repeat three more times.
16. Rest in the Child Posture (asana 16) for 60 seconds when you have completed all repetitions.

7. BOW (DHANURASANA)

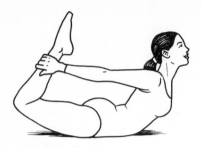

The Bow increases vitality by supplying your thyroid, parathyroid, adrenal and gonad glands with a rich supply of blood. The bow is especially recommended for people with disorders of the urinary system and prostate.

Benefits

✓ strengthens back and thigh muscles and helps align the vertebrae of the back

✓ strengthens knee joints

✓ helps to remove stagnant toxic materials from the intestinal tract because the abdominal organs are pressed against the floor

✓ improves the function of the liver, kidneys, spleen, stomach and intestines

! Do not strain the back of the neck or throat when holding this posture.

Start

1. Lie face-down on the floor with your arms beside your body and palms facing down.

Basic posture

2. Bend your knees and bring your feet toward the buttocks.

3. Without raising the chin off the floor, reach back and grip your feet or ankles.

4. Inhale and slowly raise your head, shoulders, chest and knees. If you cannot raise the knees when you start practicing this

posture, just raise the trunk until your body becomes more flexible.

Align and hold

5. Keep your feet close together as you press the legs as far away from your body as is comfortable without straining.
6. Breathe normally and allow yourself to feel the beautiful stretch across the chest. Feel your chest expanding while you hold this posture.
7. Look up without constricting the back of the neck.
8. Stretch your head away from your shoulders.
9. Allow all your body weight to rest on the abdominal area. Create resistance by pulling on the legs with your arms while you continue to press your legs away from the body.
10. Hold the posture for 30 seconds.

Release

11. Exhale, release the arms and slowly lower your legs until your knees touch the floor. Then lower your torso. Return to the starting position, relax and take three deep breaths.
12. Repeat three more times.

- Maintain a firm grip on the feet or ankles.
- Continue to press the thighs and shins away from the body.
- Feet should be raised higher than the head.
- Increase the extension of the front of the body by pressing the legs away from you; this will also increase the curve of the spine.
- Keep your feet as close together as you can.
- Lift and expand your chest.

8. BRIDGE (SETU BANDHASANA)

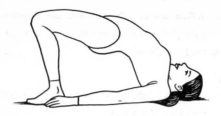

The position of the Bridge includes the chin lock, another important exercise in yoga, which improves the functioning of the thyroid and parathyroid glands. This makes the Bridge a good asana for people with problems caused by an underactive thyroid. This posture is also excellent for promoting abdominal breathing – an important component of yoga practice. It stimulates circulation in the vena cava and aorta (the main blood vessels leading to and from the heart).

Benefits

✓ promotes a healthy spine by bending it backward, opposing our natural inclination to slouch (works to eliminate hunchback, opens chest area and releases tension around the shoulders)

✓ an excellent stretch for the pancreas (people with diabetes will find this a beneficial posture)

! **Do not** practice this posture if you are pregnant. If you have high blood pressure **do not hold** the posture.

Start

1. Begin lying on your back with your arms at your side, palms facing down.

2. Bend your knees, keep your feet on the floor and bring your heels as close to the buttocks as possible. The feet should be approximately 15 cm (six inches) apart and pointing straight forward. The second toe of each foot should be aligned with the center of the knee.

3. Exhale.

Basic posture

4. As you inhale, slowly raise your pelvis and trunk as high as you can, forming a bridge.
5. Place your hands under the ribcage for support, with your fingertips pointing toward the spine. Your elbows should be as close to the body as possible.

Align and hold

6. Raise your pelvis as high as possible, pressing your shoulders and upper arms into the floor.
7. Walk the shoulder blades toward each other to lift you higher. It is important that the shoulders, not your neck, support the weight in this area.
8. You should feel an expansion in your chest as you continue to press your pelvis and trunk up. Press your chin as close to the chest as you can. Feel the vertebra in your neck being stretched.
9. Breathing is deep, slow and concentrated in the abdominal area. Your belly should feel like you are repeatedly filling and releasing air in a balloon.
10. Press your feet, especially the big toes, into the floor and move the chest closer to the chin to receive the most benefit from this posture.
11. Hold for 30 seconds.

Release

12. Release your arms from supporting your back and return them so they lie flat on the floor, palms facing down.
13. Slowly exhale and descend vertebrae by vertebrae. Feel each vertebra touch the floor as your pelvis and torso slowly return to rest on the floor.
14. When your buttocks are resting on the floor, extend your legs.
15. Relax - take three deep breaths.
16. Repeat three more times.

9. BOAT (NAVASANA)

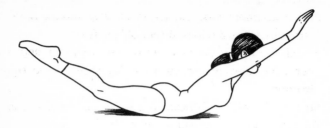

The Boat is another posture that bends the spine backward, against our natural inclination to bend forward, and that is very helpful to prevent or relieve back problems and slouching.

Benefits

✓ strengthens all of the back muscles and the entire spine

✓ improves digestion, the body's elimination of waste and the function of the vital organs

✓ If you suffer with slipped discs you may find relief by practicing this posture regularly.

! **Do not** practice this posture if you have a hiatus hernia.

Start

1. Lie face down with your forehead resting on the floor. Fully extend your arms in front of you with your thumbs touching and your palms facing down. Your legs are resting on the floor and your ankles are together.

Basic posture

2. Simultaneously lift your arms and legs off the floor, keeping them together and as straight as possible.

Align and hold

3. Take a half breath and lift the upper body and legs off the floor. Do not try to lift and breathe at the same time as you may experience cramping in the diaphragm. In the beginning you may find it difficult to lift both your chest and legs off the floor,

but this will become easier as your abdominal muscles get stronger. The pressure on the hara center stimulates the energy flow.

4. Press your pubic bone and abdominal area into the floor to lift your arms, torso and legs further off the floor.

5. Stretch the tips of your toes away from your hips and stretch your heels upward. Stretch your fingertips in the opposite direction.

6. Stretch the top of your head away from your shoulders and feel the elongation of your spine and neck.

7. Breathe normally and hold for 30 seconds.

Release

8. Exhale and slowly lower your legs and arms simultaneously.

9. Turn your head to one side.

10. Relax and take three deep breaths.

11. Repeat three more times.

10. WHEELBARROW

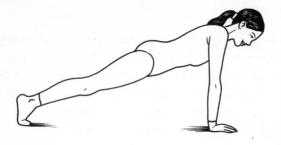

This position is very much like an extended push-up; the body forms an inclined plane. You want to maintain straight arms and a straight spine – do not allow the spine to be concave.

The emphasis in this yoga posture is to sustain it with good alignment. It is important to hold the pose without moving around or shaking. Unlike other forms of exercise, there is no concern with the number of push-ups that you can do.

Benefits
- ✓ strengthens the arms, shoulders, back, legs and feet
- ✓ stimulates circulation
- ✓ improves posture

Start
1. Lie face down on the floor with your legs together. Your toes are tucked under to provide support.
2. Place your palms flat on the floor beside your shoulders with the fingers pointing forward and slightly apart.

Basic posture
3. Take a deep breath and push your body up until your arms are straight. Only the palms of the hands, thumbs and the toes support the weight of the body.
4. Your head, spine and legs should be in a straight line. From the side, you look like an inclined plane.

Align and hold

5.   Breathe normally and hold the posture for as long as you can.

Release

6.   Exhale as you bend the arms and lower the body slowly toward the floor. If you have a weak back, bend your knees first, let them touch the floor and then lower the rest of the body. When you become more flexible, bring the knees down first, and from this position, push the buttocks back slightly, drop your chest and scoop forward, touching the chin next and slide forward until you are flat on the floor.

7.   Turn your head, lie on the floor and relax while you take three deep breaths.

8.   Repeat three more times.

11. SHOULDER STAND (SARVANGASANA)

Sarvangasana is the mother of all asanas. Just as a mother strives for harmony in the home, this asana strives for harmony in the body. *Sarvangasana* is one of the greatest boons conferred on humanity by our ancient sages.

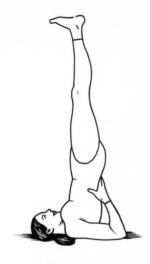

Benefits

✓ promotes blood circulation around the neck and chest (the supply of blood is regulated by the firm chin-lock position, stimulating the thyroid and parathyroid glands)

✓ promotes relief from breathlessness, palpitations, asthma, bronchitis or throat ailments

✓ inverted position good for soothing nerves and relieving headaches, colds or other nasal disturbances (also recommended for urinary disorders, uterine displacement, piles and hernia)

❗ Do not attempt the shoulder stand if you suffer from high blood pressure or severe neck problems.

Start

1. Begin by lying flat on your back. Place your hands beside the body with palms facing down. For more comfort, place a folded blanket under your upper body, shoulders and arms. Your head must remain on the floor.

Basic posture

3. Bend your legs and bring them toward the stomach.
4. Exhale and raise your hips – support them with your hands. Your knees are together and resting just above your head.

5. Take a deep breath. With the next exhalation, straighten and raise your legs so that they are perpendicular to the floor and your toes are pointed. If this is too difficult, just straighten the legs and raise them to a three-quarter position. When you are more proficient and comfortable with this move, you can stretch the legs all the way up. The back of your head, neck and shoulders and the back of the upper arms remain resting on the floor.

6. Place both hands on the back of your ribcage; the elbows should be facing straight back, approximately shoulder-width apart for the best support.

Align and hold

7. Keep pressing your hands into your back and move the chest toward the chin, keeping the legs and toes pointing straight up.

8. Hold the posture for 30 seconds.

! **Do not** hold this posture if you feel pressure in the head, ears, eyes or throat.

Release

9. To release, first bend your knees and bring them toward your forehead. If comfortable, rest the knees beside the ears, just as in the Plough.

10. Slowly release your arms from supporting the back and place them on the floor beside you.

11. Bring down your hips by slowly rolling the spine out, vertebra by vertebra; do not lift your head from the floor.

12. When your hips touch the floor, straighten your legs upward. With the next exhalation, lower your legs to the floor, with the feet together. Do not arch your back during this final phase of the release. If this is too difficult, bend your knees slightly while lowering the legs to the floor.

13. Relax on your back for three deep breaths.

14. Repeat three more times.

12. SPINAL TWIST (ARBHA MATSYENDRASANA)

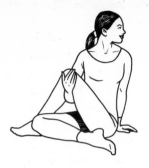

This asana is named for Matsyendra, one of the founders of hatha yoga. His story demonstrates the historical and spiritual links between yoga and the Hindu culture. One day the Hindu Lord Siva went to a deserted island with his consort, Parvati, to teach her everything there was to know about yoga. During these lessons a fish came close to the shore and, taking an interest, listened intently to all of Lord Siva's teachings.

The presence of the fish eventually became apparent to Lord Siva. Realizing that the fish had learned all the teachings of yoga, Lord Siva sprinkled water on the fish and immediately the fish gained divine form. The newly transformed fish was called Matsyendra and, in human form, he spread the knowledge of yoga for the remainder of his life.

Benefits

✓ stretches and lengthens the muscles and ligaments of the spine, keeping the spine elastic and healthy

✓ massages the spinal fluid through turning of the spine, which has a calming effect on the nervous system

✓ improves posture and mobility of the neck, thorax, waist and lower spine. An excellent stretch for sciatic nerves

! If you suffer from severe knee injuries, do this posture keeping one or both legs straight. **Do not** do this posture if you have had surgery in the previous three months. Use caution if you have fused vertebrae.

Start

1. Begin from a seated position on the floor, with both legs stretched out in front of you.

Basic posture

2. Draw your right foot close to the body, keeping the knee pointing upward.

3. Cross your right foot over the left leg, placing the sole of your foot on the ground close to the knee.

4. Bend your extended left leg, drawing the foot in close to the opposite buttock - your knee remains on the floor. If you experience too much discomfort in this position, or if both buttocks do not touch the ground, leave the left leg extended.

5. Press your buttocks into the floor. Put your left hand through the middle of the bent right leg just behind the knee. Wrap your hand around the knee and pull it as close to the body as you can.

6. Place your right hand behind your body, not so far away from the body as to cause the spine to curve or slouch.

7. Straighten and elongate your spine, keeping the spine straight so that you receive a good lateral stretch in that area.

8. Exhale and gently turn to the right (toward the bent leg), starting at the sacrum and moving up through the lumbar, mid-spine, upper spine, neck and finally turn your head as far as possible.

9. Gaze over your right shoulder, position your chin parallel to the floor and try to align the chin with the right shoulder. Look as far to the right as you can, keeping your eyes relaxed.

Align and hold

10. Consciously relax in the posture. You may notice that your breathing is faster - that is because the diaphragm is being squeezed by the spinal twist. After some practice, the pose can be held for 30 to 60 seconds with normal breathing.

11. Keep pressing your right foot into the floor while holding this posture.

Release

12. Slowly release from the posture by turning to face forward.

13. Release your arms and straighten your legs.

14. Take three deep breaths.

15. Elongate your spine and then repeat on the other side.

16. Repeat three more times.

13. LAUGHASANA

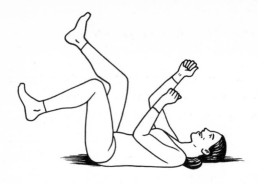

We all know that laughter is the best medicine. As you practice Laughasana, enjoy yourself.

Benefits

✓ very good for people suffering from depression, sadness, chronic negativity or grief

✓ brings additional blood, oxygen and energy to every part of the body, nourishing each cell (when we don't nourish the cells with a fresh supply of blood, oxygen and energy, they can't eliminate the toxins that lead to illness)

Start

1. Lie flat on your back.
2. Raise your legs perpendicular to the floor.

Basic posture

3. Pump your legs as though you are riding a bicycle and match that movement with your arms.
4. Make a loose fist with your hands and harmonize the action of your arms with the action of your legs.
5. Laugh as loud as you can. Engage your entire body in the laughter. Don't worry if you feel that you are pretending to laugh; eventually the laugh will be heartfelt.

Align and hold

6. Continue for three minutes.

7. Do it every day to promote good health.

Release

8. Gradually slow down and finally stop the pumping motion.
9. Lie flat on your back and breath normally for 60 seconds.
10. Repeat anytime you need an energy boost.

 Blood, oxygen and energy are naturally drawn to the hara center. Through laughing, the hara center acts as a pump and combined with the pumping action of the arms and legs, these vital elements are transported to the extremities of the body. It is not hard to feel this area moving when you laugh. After a few minutes of laughing and pumping your arms and legs, you will feel your body temperature increase and a warm current flowing through your body.

14. LION (SIMHASANA)

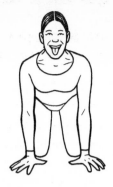

In Sanskrit, *simha* means lion. In this posture your body shape looks a growling lion. This releases tension from the neck and throat and is especially good for people who have a blockage in this area. It is said to be helpful for people who stammer.

Benefits

✓ makes the voice soft and melodious

✓ relieves and prevents sore throats

✓ relieves pain in the coccyx

✓ exercises the liver and controls the flow of life

✓ even said to cure bad breath

! If you wear dentures, exercise caution when stretching out the tongue.

Start

1. Sit in a kneeling posture, with your buttocks resting on your heels and the front of each foot resting flat on the floor.
2. Rest the palms of your hands on your knees.
3. Elongate your spine.
4. Close your eyes, take a deep complete breath and exhale with a growl. Open your eyes.

Basic posture

5. Lift your body slightly off the heels and stretch forward, maintaining a straight back.

6. Stretch the arms in front of you and place your hands on the floor, fingers spread apart. Some of your body weight is shifted to the hands.

7. Open your mouth wide. Stretch your tongue out and down toward the chin as far as you can. Stretch out your claws (fingers).

In this posture you have to do five things simultaneously: stretch forward; open your mouth wide; stretch out the tongue; roll the eyes up; and growl from the center of your being.

Align and hold

8. Gaze up toward the center of the eyebrows.

9. Hold the posture for 30 seconds while breathing through the mouth and nose.

Release

10. Withdraw the tongue into the mouth.

11. Sit back on your heels and put your hands back on your knees.

12. Close your eyes and take three deep breaths.

For relief of sore throats, stretch your tongue out and let the sun shine down your throat. The sun is considered to have disinfectant properties, which are particularly strong in the morning.

15. CAT

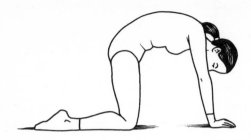

This asana is aptly named for its resemblance to the stretching routine of a cat. Cats are well known for their suppleness and ability to relax anywhere, anytime – one of the goals of any yoga practitioner.

Benefits
- ✓ helps in management of hypertension
- ✓ limbers the spinal column and relieves tension in the lower spine
- ✓ corrects tense breathing patterns
- ✓ aids digestion by encouraging peristaltic action of material through the digestive tract
- ✓ used in prenatal and postnatal exercises (helps the uterus return to normal position after childbirth)
- ✓ provides a natural massage for stomach, intestines, colon, liver, kidneys, gallbladder and pancreas
- **!** **Do not** pull your abdomen so close to the spine if you are pregnant.

Start
1. Kneel on all fours with your palms directly beneath the shoulders; arms are straight. The knees are aligned with the hips.
2. Press your weight into the palms of your hands and into your shins.
3. Stretch your tailbone away from your hip and stretch the crown of your head away from your shoulders. Feel the elongation of your spine.

4. Arms should be locked and vertical. The back should be parallel to the floor. Your neck and head are in line with the back. This position is also called the Table Posture.

Basic posture

5. Breathe in slowly and deeply, arching your back and looking up.
6. Exhale completely and round your spine upward – bending it in the opposite direction – like an abdominal lift. The exhalation makes it possible for you to pull your abdomen in toward the spine.
7. Drop your head and tuck the chin toward your chest. Drop your tailbone down as your curl your spine.

Align and hold

8. Repeat steps 5, 6 and 7 three times without stopping – breathing deeply and smoothly. Don't hold either the concave or the arched stretch – coordinate your breath with the movement of the spine.
9. Rest in the starting position (Table Posture) for five to 10 seconds.

Release

10. Repeat three more times.
11. Relax in the Child Posture (asana 16) for three deep breaths.

Variation

• While still in the Table Posture, slowly stretch out your right leg and left arm, keeping both parallel to the floor.
• Stretch your head forward.
• Hold this posture for 30 seconds, breathing normally.
• Slowly release and repeat on the other side.
• Repeat three more times on each side.
• After you have done three of these, exhale slowly. Then lower your head and bend your right knee, bringing it as close as possible to the forehead, while you arch your back upward with a stretch. Take one deep breath into this stretch and release – repeat on the other side.
• Relax into the Child Posture.

16. CHILD POSTURE (BALASANA)

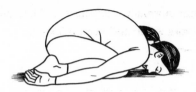

Psychologically this asana implies surrender – of your ego or egotism. It means letting go of the state of mind that boasts, "I know," also letting go of greed, jealousy, anger and all other negative emotions associated with egotism.

Benefits

✓ relieves strain and pain in the lower back
✓ relaxes the back and promotes healing of serious injuries
✓ takes pressure away from the intervertebral discs
✓ improves digestion
✓ removes tension from neck and shoulders
❗ **Do not** hold this posture if you have high blood pressure. Exercise caution if you have knee problems – do not practice if you feel pain in the knees.

Start

1. Begin in a kneeling position, with your knees slightly apart to prevent compressing the hara center. The buttocks rest on your heels, and the top of your feet should be flat on the floor. Your spine is straight and your arms are relaxed at your sides.

Basic posture

2. Inhale and elongate your spine.
3. Exhale and slowly stretch forward. Begin by tilting the hips forward first and keep stretching forward until your stomach and chest rests on your thighs. Let your forehead rest on the floor in front of your knees.

4. Keep your arms straight back and relaxed at your side, palms facing up.

Align and hold

5. As you breathe normally, feel your shoulders drop closer to the ground and your spine and neck relaxing.
6. Hold for 30 seconds.

If at first you cannot rest your forehead on the floor, do not raise your buttocks off your heels. Continue to elongate the spine throughout the posture. Stretch your head away from the shoulders and eventually your forehead will reach the floor.

Release

7. Inhale, release and come up to the starting position.
8. Take three deep breaths.
9. Repeat three more times.

If you tend to be inflexible, you may not find this posture to be restful at first. To make it easier, spread the knees farther apart, especially if you are overweight. Rest your fists, one on top of the other, on the floor in front of your knees to provide an elevated platform to rest your forehead on. Try to find the adaptation of this pose that is most comfortable for you, then remain still.

17. THIGH STRETCH (LUNGE)

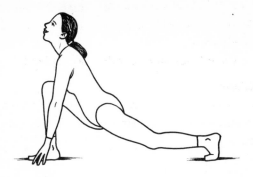

The Lunge (Hanumanasana) is an excellent stretch for the groin. It brings blood into the pelvic area and tones the abdominal organs.

Benefits
✓   strengthens the legs, arms and back, especially the muscles around the knees

✓   a good stretch for the Achilles tendon and hamstring muscles making this a good posture for runners' warm-up routines. (Also recommended to relieve cramps in the calf and thigh muscles.)

!   **Do not** practice the lunge if you are suffering from injuries to ligaments, Achilles tendon or hamstrings.

Start
1. Start from the Mountain Pose (asana 19).
2. Take three deep breaths and let all your weight be supported by the earth.
3. Exhale and take a long step forward with your right leg.

Basic posture
4. Bend both knees so that you can rest your hands on either side of your front foot, approximately shoulder-width apart.
5. The back knee should be about 5 cm (two inches) off the ground, with your toes tucked under the foot. The front knee should not extend past the middle toe of the foot.

6. Look forward and up.
7. Exhale and straighten both legs while keeping your hands on the floor. Your back heel should be pressing into the floor and your head should be pointing toward the floor with your back stretched down.
8. Repeat three times on each side – do not hold.

Align and hold
9. The center of your front knee should be aligned with the toe next to the big toe. (This strengthens the muscles around the patella.)

Release
10. Repeat three times on each side, then release.
11. Bend both knees, keeping your hands on the floor.
12. Lower your back knee to two inches off the ground. As you release, exhale and drop the back knee to the floor.
13. Align your front knee with the back – now both knees are resting on the floor.
14. Lower the rest of the body to the floor, turn the head to one side and rest. Take three deep breaths.
15. Repeat with the other leg.

18. SQUATTING POSTURE (UTKATASANA)

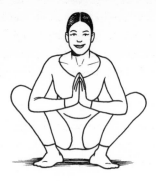

Utkata means powerful, fierce and uneven. This asana is like sitting on an imaginary stool. This is one of the most important asanas in hatha yoga. Most Westerners do this move incorrectly by lifting their heels. To strengthen your ankles, it is necessary to perform this posture flat-footed.

Benefits

✓ good for prostate problems if practiced on the toes – but first it must be mastered by keeping the feet flat on the floor

✓ excellent for reducing menstrual problems, particularly cramps

✓ strengthens legs and releases pressure from the lower spine

✓ provides a gentle massage for the heart as the diaphragm is lifted

✓ assists in the body's elimination process by stimulating the peristaltic movement of materials through the digestive tract

! Exercise caution with this posture if you have knee problems. Improper alignment of your knees can create additional problems. The center of the knee needs to be aligned with the toe next to the big toe in this posture. This usually requires you to continually press the thighs outward.

Start

1. Stand with your feet 30 to 40 cm (12 to 18 inches) apart. Your feet are slightly angled outward depending on what is comfortable for you. Balance your weight equally on both feet. Ground yourself by focusing on the connection between your feet and the earth. Feel pressure on all nine points of each foot.

There are nine points on the sole of your foot that you need to become aware of when doing this posture:

- the soft pad of each toe
- two soft balls or pads of the front of the foot
- soft ball or pad of the heel
- outer edge of the back three-quarters of your foot

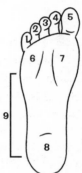

Basic posture

2. Exhale and lower your buttocks to the floor as low as you can, depending on your flexibility.
3. Press the palms of your hands together so there is force in the arms.
4. Ensure the centers of the knees are aligned with the toe next to the big toe – this cannot be emphasized enough. You can place your elbows inside of the upper thighs to press your legs outward for proper alignment.
5. Keep your spine as straight as possible by keeping the chest as far back as possible. Try not to slouch forward.

Press your feet into the floor feeling all nine points of the foot connecting to the ground. If you have balance problems you can stretch the arms straight out, and if you need extra balance to keep from lifting your heels off the floor, you can hold onto a steady object, like a door frame or heavy chair.

Align and hold

6. Relax your abdomen and breathe deeply. You should feel your abdomen pressing against the thighs each time you inhale.
7. Give yourself permission to let go of any tension in your lower spine and feel the spine elongating as you stretch the crown of your head upwards.
8. Hold for 30 seconds.

Release

9. Feel the floor with your feet and push yourself up slowly from the soles of your feet.
10. Keep your head down as you stand up. After you are fully upright – lift your head. This will prevent dizziness.
11. Repeat three more times.

Variation

In addition to the other benefits of the Squatting Posture, you can get an excellent workout for your heart, increase blood circulation and help prevent prolapse with this variation. Repeat it without stopping, slowly moving up and down 12 times. This requires a lot of stamina, but if you practice it regularly you will develop the stamina you need to increase the number of repetitions. Use this variation of the Squatting Posture when lifting heavy objects to prevent spinal damage.

•   From the standing position with your feet pointed out at a 45-degree angle, exhale, then bend your knees and lower the buttocks as far as your flexibility permits, without touching the floor. (Imagine you have a chair behind you and follow your body's natural alignment as if you are going to sit down.)

- Do not hunch forward. You can lean forward, but keep your back straight.
- Your arms are outstretched in front of you with palms facing the floor. Turn your palms up each time you stand up and turn the palms down each time you go down. As you go up and down, let your arms lead slightly, almost like they are pulling you up and pushing you down. Keep the speed of your descent and ascent moderate.
- It is very important to keep the middle of your knees properly aligned with the second toe throughout.
- Do 12 repetitions, slowly. (One repetition is a complete up and down motion.)
- Rest in the Mountain Pose (asana 19) with your eyes closed. Breathe deeply, and as soon as you can, drop the breath down to the hara center.
- After one week of practicing this every day, increase the number of repetitions to 20 or 25.

19. MOUNTAIN POSE (TADASANA)

Learning to stand correctly is an essential element of yoga and many other forms of intense bodywork. Most kung fu schools include the Mountain Pose to teach students correct posture and proper alignment of the entire body from head to toe. *Tadasana* is a powerful working posture that reduces wear and tear on the body if incorporated into your everyday life. You can check your posture by standing beside a full-length mirror – a straight line should run through the ear, shoulder, hip, knee and anklebone

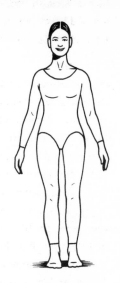

Tada means mountain. Most people stand without distributing their body weight evenly on their feet. Improper weight distribution can lead to specific problems. For instance, if you stand with your body weight back on the heels, the effect of gravity changes the body. The hips become loose, the abdomen protrudes, the body hangs back and strain is put on the spine. Standing too erect and slouching forward both create strain on your spine. Refer to the key point in the Squatting Posture (asana 18) that describes the nine points of the feet – your weight should be on all these points to attain proper weight distribution.

When your body is not aligned, your organs are not aligned. This impedes the proper function of the internal organs and also blocks the flow of energy in the body.

Benefits
- ✓   strengthens a weak body structure
- ✓   helps reduce back problems and headaches caused by carrying the head too far forward
- ✓   improves spinal alignment, circulation and breathing
- ✓   tones leg muscles
- ✓   increases body awareness and gives a sense of being balanced, centered and grounded

Start
1. Stand straight with your feet facing straight ahead. Women should have their feet 5 cm (two inches) apart and men should have their big toes and ankles lightly touching.

Basic posture
2. Firmly connect each of the nine points of your foot (taught in the Squatting Posture) to the ground.
3. Toes are relaxed and slightly spaced apart – do not grip the floor with your toes.
4. Knees are soft, not rigid, and the center of the knee is aligned with the second toe. To check, look down at your toes and bend your knees until you can see the tips of your toes just beyond the knee. Now align the center of your knees with the toe next to the big toe and pull your knees back while maintaining this alignment. Do not hyperextend your knees – they should remain soft.
5. Arms are relaxed at your side with your palms facing the thighs. Create a little space under the armpits.
6. Create space between your thighs by pressing them outward to counter the normal tendency to sag inwards. This will shift more of your weight to the outer edge of the feet. As you become more proficient in this posture, your weight will become more equally distributed.

Align and hold
7. Elongate your spine making yourself taller without creating tension in the shoulder area. Feel an expansion in your chest.
8. Stretch your head away from your shoulders with the chin slightly down to reduce pressure on your neck.
9. The overall feeling should be that of natural firmness and poise.
10. Relax the muscles of the face and eyes. Look straight ahead.

Release
11. Hold the posture for 60 seconds while you breathe deeply into the abdominal area, focusing on the hara center (Chapter 1). Do not lift up the chest as you inhale.

20. CLASSICAL FORWARD STRETCH (PADAHASTASANA)

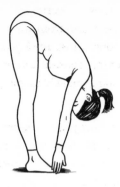

In Sanskrit, *pada* means foot and *hasta* means hand. This is a relaxing posture that provides a passive elongation and stretch for your body. Poor posture and tension restrict the flow of blood and energy to the neck and shoulder area. This asana counters these restrictions and relieves discomfort in this area.

Benefits

✓ increases the suppleness of the spine by stretching it
✓ strengthens and tones the legs
✓ provides a good stretch for the hamstrings
✓ nourishes tissues of the face and scalp with an additional supply of blood
✓ helps decrease fat in the abdominal area
! **Do not hold** this posture if you have high or low blood pressure.

Start

1. Stand with your feet approximately 30 cm (12 inches) apart. The feet should be angled slightly outwards. If you have sciatic nerve problems, have the toes pointing slightly toward each other. Your arms rest at your side.

Basic posture

2. Inhale and raise your arms out from the sides in a semicircle until they reach over the head. Align arms beside your ears; palms face forward.

3. The idea of this posture is to stretch the spine, not just bend it. So it is very important to stretch up, elongating the spine and creating space between the vertebrae.

4. Exhale and stretch forward from the hips, keeping your head aligned between your arms, until your arms and head are hanging straight down. Maintain a strong stretch in your arms to help keep your spine straight as you go forward and down.

Align and hold

5. Depending on your suppleness, grasp your toes, ankles or calves, to pull your body closer to the thighs.

6. Consciously relax and let go of tension in your abdomen, shoulders, neck and head.

7. Hold for 30 seconds while breathing normally. Focusing your breathing into the hara center will help relax your lower back.

 Keep your feet firmly attached to the floor and the legs straight. In the down position, lengthen the front of your body and the spine toward the floor, while stretching the head toward the floor to release pressure from the neck vertebrae. Keep your abdomen relaxed and bring it as close to the thighs as possible.

Release

8. Release the arms and stretch them forward as you inhale and slowly come back up, continuing to keep the spine straight. Come up in the same manner you went down, with your arms stretched out and your head aligned between them. Keep your chin slightly tucked down and lift your head last to prevent dizziness. If you have back problems, curl your back as you come up.

9. When you are upright, with your arms stretched above you, exhale and lower the arms in a semicircle to the side.

10. Take three deep breaths, and repeat three more times.

21. BACK BEND (URDHVASANA)

The Classical Forward Stretch complements the Back Bend and these two asanas should be done together. Start with the Classical Forward Stretch and when you are in the upright position, always take three deep breaths before commencing with the Back Bend. This is to allow the equilibrium in your ears to return to normal.

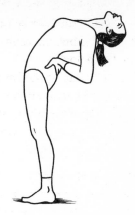

Benefits

✓   good posture to reverse and prevent rounded shoulders and hunched backs

✓   improves the flow of blood, oxygen and energy to the nerves of the spine

✓   stretches the pancreas, making this a very helpful asana for diabetics

!   **Do not** attempt this asana if you suffer from dizziness.

!   If your spine starts to quiver while doing this posture, release yourself. This simply means that your spine is not strong enough to hold the posture, or you have stretched back too far.

Start

1. Start with the Classical Forward Stretch. When you return to the upright position, take three deep breaths before starting the Back Stretch.

2. Stand as you would in the Mountain Pose (asana 19), only with the feet approximately 30 cm (12 inches) apart. Your toes are pointing straight ahead, or can be slightly turned out. You may want to place your hands on the mid-back for support; fingers point toward the spine.

Basic posture

3. Inhale, lift your ribcage without moving your pelvis and elongate your spine. This will create more space between the vertebrae to allow you to stretch a little further with more comfort.

4. Look up at the ceiling and stretch the front of your neck.

5. Exhale and let the shoulders fall back naturally.

6. Without pushing the hips forward, slowly stretch backward from the waist without straining. Use common sense to know when you have reached the limit of your flexibility.

Align and hold

7. Gently tighten the buttocks.

8. Do not hold the muscles in tension, but consciously let go and allow your shoulders to drop back a little further. You should feel your chest opening up and expanding.

9. Breathe deeply into the abdominal area.

10. Hold for 10 to 30 seconds.

 Stay firmly connected to the floor with your feet. The muscles of your back should remain soft. Remember that the extension of the spine should be even. Do not lean to one side or the other. Keep the front of your throat stretched and **do not** bend the knees.

Release

11. Do not jerk forward when releasing this posture. Slowly come forward from the waist, using the strength of your legs to steady you.

12. Take three deep breaths to allow the equilibrium in your ears to return to normal.

13. Follow with another Classical Forward Bend.

22. TRIANGLE (TRIKONASANA)

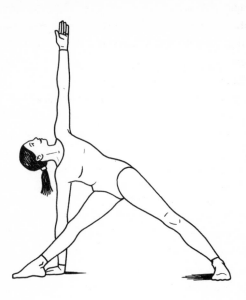

Tri means three and *kona* means angle. The *Trikonasana* teaches alignment and a sense of direction by creating several triangles within the posture.

Benefits

- ✓ removes superfluous fat from the waist and hips
- ✓ expands and opens the chest area
- ✓ stretches the arms, shoulders, back, legs and internal organs – especially the lungs
- ✓ nourishes the nerves of the spine with extra blood
- ✓ corrects minor deformities in the legs, knees and hips, allowing them to develop evenly (as well as strengthening these areas)
- ✓ brings extra blood, oxygen and energy into the shoulder area
- ! **Do not** hold the posture if you have problems with high blood pressure. If you have problems with balance, do not stretch too low.

Start

1. Stand with your legs apart, approximately the same distance as the length of your leg.
2. Turn the right foot out to 90 degrees; the whole leg turns as well. Align the right knee with your right foot to avoid hyperextension of the knee.
3. Turn the left foot and leg inward 15 degrees.
4. Firmly press the soles of your feet into the ground.
5. Stretch the top of your head away from the shoulders and feel the elongation through your spine.
6. Stretch your arms out to the side, feeling the elongation from the sternum and spine to the fingertips of your outstretched hands, keeping the fingers together.

Basic posture

7. Press your left hip out - allowing the pressure to extend the left side of your torso. Stretch from the waist.
8. Exhale, while stretching the right arm away from the body and down toward the right foot. At the same time your left arm stretches up to be perpendicular to the floor. Maintain the stretch in the left arm from the fingertips to the shoulder.
9. Keep your right hipbone aligned with the right knee and the right foot.
10. Press your left hipbone back and up.

Align and hold

11. Rotate your chest to align your torso with the legs and hips.
12. Turn your head to look up at your left thumb.
13. Relax into this stretch and breathe normally.
14. Hold for 30 seconds.

Release

15. Press the soles of your feet into the ground. Inhale and slowly release the stretch, returning to the upright starting position the same way you went down.
16. Exhale as you bring your arms down to the side of the body.
17. Take three deep breaths, centering yourself by focusing on your breathing.
18. Repeat on the opposite side.

23. WARRIOR (VIRABHADRASANA)

The story of Vira-bhadra, one of the heroes of Hindu legend, is told by Talidasa in his great poem *Kumara Samhava* (The Birth of the Warlord). The story starts with Daksa celebrating a great sacrifice. To this sacrifice Daksa invites many gods and priests, but does not invite his daughter, Sati, or her husband, Siva, the chief of the gods. In spite of being overlooked by her father, Sati attends the sacrifice but feels insulted and greatly humiliated. As a result, Sati throws herself on the fire and perishes. When Siva hears of this, he is so angry that he tears a matted lock of hair from his head and throws it on the ground. From this lock of hair a powerful warrior arises, Virabhadra. Virabhadra leads Siva's army into battle, beheading Daksa and the gods and priests who were in attendance at the sacrifice. This asana is dedicated to the powerful hero that Siva created from a matted lock of his hair to avenge the death of his love.

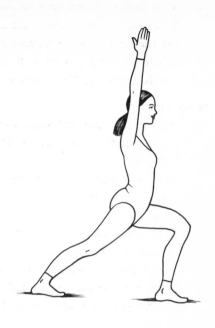

Benefits

✓ reduces fat in the hip area and firms the muscles of the stomach

✓ improves balance, concentration and alignment

✓ helps you stand firmly on the soles of the feet, making you feel grounded

! Most standing postures are strenuous, especially this one. If you have a weak heart, stretch the arms straight out from your shoulders or leave them at the side of the body when doing this asana.

Start

1. Start with the Mountain Pose (asana 19).
2. Inhale, raise your arms overhead, bringing the palms close together and facing each other at the apex.
3. Exhale and take a long step to the side – the approximate length of your leg (35 inches or one metre).

Basic posture

4. Turn to the right and simultaneously turn your right foot 90 degrees to the right and the left foot 45 degrees also to the right.
5. Bend your right knee until the right thigh is parallel with the floor and the shin is perpendicular to the floor, making a right angle with the leg.
6. Align the center of the bent knee with the second toe to strengthen the knee.
7. Stretch the left leg and turn the thigh slightly outward.
8. Relax into the right groin and turn the left hip forward and towards your bent knee as much as you can.

Align and hold

9. Your shoulders and hips should be aligned facing the right foot.
10. Elongate the spine and stretch right up to your fingertips.
11. Press the soles of your feet firmly into the ground and extend the crown of your head away from your shoulders.
12. Push forward with your back leg and backward with your front leg. Your body weight should be centered and remain still when holding this posture.
13. Breathe deeply into the hara center and hold for 30 seconds.

Release

14. Exhale, release your arms and return to the starting position with both legs straight and both feet facing forward.
15. Take three deep, relaxing breaths and repeat on the other side.

24. TREE (VRKASANA)

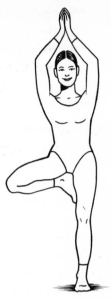

This is a focused and concentrated asana that will help you empty and still your mind. Practice the tree before you start a stressful day at the office, prior to an exam or any time you need to focus your mind and stop the onslaught of distracting random thoughts. The effect of the tree is like sending your mind on vacation. With no additional effort, the mind empties itself while you hold the posture.

Benefits

✓   tones leg, back and chest muscles

✓   strengthens ankles

✓   improves balance

!   If you have problems with dizziness or poor balance, stand near or against a wall or large heavy object when doing the Tree.

Start

1. Start with the Mountain Pose (asana 19). Take three deep breaths and center yourself.
2. Fix your gaze on a single point in front of you, level with your eyes. Shift your weight to your left leg. The knee is loose and soft (very slightly bent as opposed to rigid and hyper-extended).
3. Extend your left arm straight out to the side to provide additional balance.

Basic posture

4. Bend your right knee and grasp the ankle to bring the heel of the right foot up as high as you can to rest on the inner, upper left leg. The right leg is bent out to the side, aligned with the right hip (if possible).
5. Extend your right arm out to the side and turn both palms up. Stretch both arms out to the side (right to the fingertips).

6. Raise your arms, bringing your fingertips together over the head. Your elbows are slightly bent, but should remain aligned with the ears. The tips of each finger and the thumb of your left hand softly touch the corresponding fingers and thumb on your right hand. If you cannot easily bring your hands together over your head, just keep the arms stretched out to the side as in step 5.

Align and hold

7. Open the thigh of the bent leg outward and keep the big toe facing toward the floor. The bent knee should form at least a 90 degree angle.
8. Elongate your spine and stretch the crown of your head toward the ceiling away from your shoulders. Do not lift the shoulders or the chin.
9. Maintain your gaze straight ahead and visualize a large tree in your mind. This will help you maintain your balance.
10. Do not hold your breath; breathe deeply from the abdominal area, as you would in the abdominal breath.
11. Hold for 30 seconds.

Release

12. Exhale as you release and lower your arms.
13. Grasp the right ankle to bring the foot away from the left leg and slowly lower your right leg.
14. Center and ground yourself and repeat on the right leg.
15. Take three deep breaths. Center and ground yourself before you repeat three more times on each leg.

25. EASY POSTURE (SUKHASANA – LOTUS POSTURE)

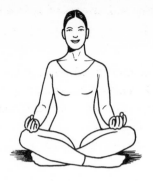

This is an important posture to learn and incorporate into your everyday life. Teach it to your children and practice it until you can hold it for a long time, like when you are reading a book, watching TV or listening to music.

Benefits

✓   strengthens spine

✓   increases flow of blood and energy through the organs

✓   prevents your organs from sagging within the abdomen

✓   exercises the muladhara chakra (the first energy center, located at the base of the spine), prostate gland and gonads

✓   creates a peaceful, still mind and body

❗   If you have knee problems **only** do this posture sitting on a chair.

Start

This posture can be done sitting cross-legged on the floor, kneeling with your feet tucked under you or sitting on a straight-backed chair (sit toward the front of the chair with your feet flat on the floor; do not lean back). To attain the most benefit from this asana, ensure that your spine is straight. In the beginning, you can sit on a firm cushion or folded blanket. As your legs become more flexible and your groin opens up, you can progress to sitting directly on the floor.

1. Sit with your head, neck and spine poised in a straight line.
2. Tuck your left foot beneath the right knee and your right foot beneath the left knee. Draw your feet in as close to the body as is comfortable.

Basic posture

3. Rest the back of each hand on its corresponding knee and touch the thumb gently to the index finger.
4. Keep your attention on your abdominal breathing and maintaining a straight spine.
5. Breathe deeply into the hara center.

Align and hold

6. Elongate your spine without creating tension by stretching your head away from your shoulders.
7. Open up your shoulders and feel your chest expanding.
8. Keep your chin slightly down to release pressure from the neck.
9. Hold for three minutes.

- There should be a straight line from your nose to your navel.
- Keep both sides of your body parallel.
- Feel your sacrum – where the base of your spine meets your pelvis – pulling downward while the rest of the spine stretches upward.
- Feel your knees getting closer to the floor with each exhalation.

Release

10. Uncross your legs and switch to the other side by placing the right foot beneath the left knee and the left foot beneath the right knee.
11. Repeat three more times and then rest by stretching the legs straight out in front of you.

CHAPTER FIVE

Yoga programs to suit your needs

PROGRAM A: TO START YOUR DAY AND ENERGIZE YOUR MIND AND BODY

Start every day by first drinking a glass of warm water to cleanse your internal system.

1. Total Relaxation Posture (asana 1) – 5 minutes

- Combine with the complete breath; work on this breath for the first three minutes.
- Select one to three affirmations and repeat three times.
- Continue to scan your body for additional tension and release it by giving yourself permission to enter a deeper and deeper level of relaxation.

2. Assorted stretching exercises

These are some simple stretching exercises that you can do to limber up your body prior to yoga practice and prevent injury. In the morning, the body is stiff and the mind is alert. It is important to bring the two into balance.

Lower spine stretch

- Lie down on your back. Keep your chin slightly toward your chest to release tension from your neck.
- With your hands, pull your right knee toward your chest. (If you have knee problems place your hands behind the knee; otherwise place your hands below the knee.)
- Push your right heel out, pointing your toes toward your head – this provides a better stretch for the back of the leg.

- Lift your left leg 2.5 to 5 cm (one to two inches) off the floor and push the heel out. You should feel an opposing stretch in each leg.
- Take three deep breaths into this stretch and release.
- Repeat with the left leg.
- Relax and take three deep breaths.

Body curl
- Remain on your back and pull both knees toward the chest.
- Align your feet and push out both heels.
- If you have no neck problems, raise your head toward the knees – curling yourself into a ball. If you have neck problems allow your head to remain on the floor.
- Breathe normally and relax into this stretch.
- You can also rock gently from side to side or back and forth if it feels comfortable for you.
- Release, relax and take three deep breaths.

Lotus Stretch
- While still on your back, bend the right leg and weave your right hand over the inner thigh and under the calf. Take hold of the calf with this hand.
- Take hold of your right heel with the left hand.
- Gently pull your bent leg horizontally toward the chest, feeling the stretch in the groin. The left leg should be 5 cm (two inches) off the floor with the heel stretched out (as in the lower spine stretch).
- Take three deep breaths into the stretch and release.
- Repeat with the left leg.
- Relax with three deep breaths.

Dancing star
- Lie on your back, with your arms resting beside the body. You can also place your hands on the hips to ensure they do not lift off the floor during this exercise.
- Lift your right knee toward your chest. With the knee, make three large circles, first in one direction and then in the opposite direction.
- Repeat with your left leg.

- After you have completed the dancing star, relax, take three deep breaths and come up to a sitting position.

3. *Back Stretch (asana 3)*
- Repeat three times.

4. *Spread Leg Stretch (asana 2)*
- Repeat three times.
- While still sitting on the floor with your spine straight, take three deep relaxing breaths.
- Come up into the Mountain Pose (asana 19) and prepare yourself for the Sun Salutation (below).

5. *Sun salutation (Surya Namashara)*
This is a complete yoga program in itself and a complete calisthenic workout. The sun salutation aids the transition our bodies must make from inactive (sleeping) to active (awake). Traditionally this program is performed at sunrise when the air is rich in *prana* – the morning is when this cosmic energy is strongest. *Surya* means sun – *namashas* means salutations.

The sun salutation is comprised of 12 positions, including seven asanas. Because of the number and repetition of postures, the benefits of the surya namahara are numerous.

Basics for the sun salutation
You should move gracefully from one position to the next, in perfect co-ordination – the program should be flowing. First become familiar with each of the movements. After that, co-ordinate your breathing with each body movement. From position 3 to position 10, it is important that your hands do not move. In the beginning, make some slight modifications, to help you move smoothly from one position to the next and to work within your physical limitations. It is important to accept limitations and not force any of the positions.

Sun salutation position 1

Mountain Posture (asana 19): Start in this position with your hands placed palms together (as if praying) in front of the chest. Your thumb should touch the heart center as a reminder of your true divinity.Close your eyes for a few seconds and concentrate on your breathing.Mentally repeat the affirmation "I open my heart to the sun." Feel the petals of your heart chakra opening in response to the warmth of the sun and the love in your heart.

Sun salutation position 2

Back Bend (asana 21): Inhale, raise your arms overhead until they are aligned with the ears, arch the spine and stretch back. (Refer to Chapter 4 for full details.)

Sun salutation position 3

Exhale and stretch forward into the Classical Forward Stretch (asana 20). Do not rise up; place the palms of your hands on the floor on either side of your feet. If you cannot comfortably reach the palms to the floor, support yourself with your fingertips.

Sun salutation position 4

Inhale and stretch the right leg back, the left foot remains between your hands.

Arch the back and look up and forward. Your body should be in a graceful curve from the head to the tip of the right foot. Refer to the Thigh Stretch (asana 17).

Sun salutation position 5

Refer to the Wheelbarrow (asana 10) and step back with your left leg so that both feet are side by side behind you with the toes curled under. Your arms should remain straight. This is the only position where the breath is held.

Sun salutation position 6

This is a transition position, not a posture. Exhale and drop both knees simultaneously to the floor, followed by the chest. Tuck in your chin and place your forehead on the floor. In this position, only the toes, knees, hands, chest and forehead touch the floor.

Sun salutation position 7

Refer to the Cobra (asana 4).

Inhale and slowly brush along the floor with your forehead, nose and chin and finally stretch the head forward and upward until you are in the Cobra.

Sun salutation position 8

Without repositioning the hands, come up into the Dog (asana 6).

Sun salutation position 9

Inhale and return to position 4 by taking a long step forward with the right foot, aligning it between the hands. At the same time, let your left knee drop to a couple of inches (4 to 6 cm) above the floor. If you cannot bring the right foot between your hands, step forward as far as you can and modify it by bringing the hands back on either side of the foot and slide the left knee back to bring you back to position 4. This modification will assist you in the beginning.

Sun salutation position 10

Exhale and return to position 3 by placing your left foot beside the right foot and straightening your legs. Your hands remain on the floor.

Sun salutation position 11

Inhale and return to position 2, slowly stretching the arms out and up until you are in the upright position, arms above your head.

Sun salutation position 12

Exhale. Return to position 1, the Mountain Pose (asana 19).

Take three deep breaths, focusing on your hara center.

Repeat the 12 positions, stepping back first with the left leg in position 4 and stepping forward first with the left leg in position 9. When completed with both legs, this is a full cycle of the sun salutation. When you are just starting out, complete two cycles only. Gradually add two more each week until you reach seven cycles. Maintain seven cycles.

Sun salutation reference page

Mountain Posture	Back bend	Forward Stretch
Inhale and stretch	Wheelbarrow	Exhale, drop knees to floor.
Cobra	Dog	Inhale and stretch
Forward stretch	Back bend	Mountain Posture

You can skip to the Total Relaxation Posture (asana 1) and end the morning program here or you can continue with the next three asanas:

6. **Spinal Twist** (asana 12)
7. **Triangle** (asana 22)
8. **Warrior** (asana 23)
9. **Total Relaxation Posture** (asana 1)

- Combine with the complete breath; work on this breath for the first three minutes.
- Select one to three affirmations and repeat three times.
- Continue to scan the body for additional tension and release it by giving yourself permission to enter a deeper and deeper level of relaxation.
- Total elapsed time for this posture, 5 minutes.

PROGRAM B: TO END YOUR DAY AND RELEASE TENSION

In the evening, the body is more flexible, but the mind is tired. The evening program will bring both into balance.

Begin and end as in the morning program, but stay in the Total Relaxation Posture (asana 1) for 12 to 15 minutes. Follow the number of repetitions indicated in Chapter 4 for each asana.

Program format

1. **Total Relaxation Posture** – 12 to 15 minutes
2. **Assorted stretching exercises** (refer to morning program)
3. **Back Stretch** (asana 3)
4. **Spread Leg Stretch** (asana 2)
5. **Cobra** (asana 4)
6. **Dog** (asana 6)
7. **Boat** (asana 9)
8. **Wheelbarrow** (asana 10)
9. **Child Posture** (asana 16)
10. **Bridge** (asana 8)
11. **Bow** (asana 7)
12. **Plough** (asana 5)
13. **Shoulder Stand** (asana 11)
14. **Cat** (asana 15)
15. **Spinal Twist** (asana 12)

16. **Thigh Stretch** (asana 17)
17. **Easy Posture** (asana 25)
18. **Squatting Posture** (asana 18)
19. **Mountain Pose** (asana 19)
20. **Classical Forward Stretch** (asana 20)
21. **Back Bend** (asana 21)
22. **Triangle** (asana 22)
23. **Warrior** (asana 23)
24. **Tree** (asana 24)
25. **Total Relaxation Posture** – 12 to 15 minutes

If you do not have enough time to complete all of these asanas, start with the first two, then choose four or five other asanas from the list and complete the program with the Total Relaxation Posture for 2 to 15 minutes.

If you stretch the spine in one direction, it is advisable to also stretch it in the opposite direction. This is why the Classical Forward Stretch and the Back Bend are done in sequence.

PROGRAM C: FOR QUICK STRESS REDUCTION

These are asanas and exercises that are modified so you can do them while in the office, without causing too much distraction to those around you. The modern workplace is one of our most stressful places, so try taking a yoga break at least once in the morning and once in the afternoon. You will find that you will be more relaxed and able to work more efficiently after a short, effective break.

1. **Modified Spinal Twist**
- Refer to the Spinal Twist (asana 12).
- Sit up straight in your chair, with your feet firmly placed on the ground in front of you.
- Inhale and place your right hand on the outside of your left knee.

- Exhale as you slowly turn to the left. Start with your head and progress to the waist.
- Place your left hand on the back or side of the chair of the chair.
- Look as far over your left shoulder as you can. Try to align your chin with your shoulder.
- Take three deep breaths and repeat on the other side.
- Repeat three more times on each side.

2. *Modified Child Posture*
Refer to the Child Posture (asana 16) for benefits and details.
- Sit straight up in your chair, feet together and flat on the floor.
- Inhale and elongate your spine by stretching your head up without lifting the shoulders.
- Exhale as you stretch forward and wrap your arms around your knees. Your stomach and chest should rest on your thighs.
- Drop your head and let it hang over the knees.
- Take three deep, slow breaths.
- Repeat three more times.

3. *Complete breath*
Refer to Chapter 2 for details. Practice this any time you are feeling stressed, overwhelmed, angry or frustrated.

Practice for one to three minutes sitting straight up in a chair.
- Close your eyes, relax and center yourself. Exhale completely.
- Slowly inhale through the nose to a count of four, filling first the abdomen, then the intercostal area and finally the upper lungs. Do not raise your shoulders up at any time during this breath. Each of the three areas should be filled with one third of the total breath.
- Exhale to the count of four, reversing the order of the inhalation. Your goal is to empty the upper region, middle region and, finally, abdominal region of the lungs.
- Squeeze out as much stale air as possible by collapsing the abdomen so it becomes concave and pulling the diaphragm muscle up under the ribcage.

4. **Abdominal breath**

   Refer to Chapter 2 for details.

5. **Seated knee squeeze**
   - Sit upright in your chair, feet flat on the floor.
   - Raise your right knee and grasp it with both hands.
   - Gently pull your knee toward you, keeping the toe pointed downward.
   - Breathe into this stretch three times.
   - Repeat on the other side.
   - Repeat both sides three times.

6. **Standing reach**
   - Stand in the the Mountain Posture (asana 19).
   - Fix your gaze on a single spot for balance.
   - Inhale as you raise your arms in a wide circle out to the side as you simultaneously come up on your toes. Place your hands palms together above your head.
   - As you complete your inhalation, co-ordinate the breath, arms and feet so your hands are just coming together over your head when you are as far up on your toes as you can be.
   - Stretch a little further toward the ceiling.
   - Exhale as you return to the starting position, co-ordinating the breath with your arms and feet.
   - Repeat three times.

7. **Elbow touch**
   - Stand in the Mountain Pose (asana 19), or sit straight in your chair.
   - Bend your elbow and rest your fingers on your shoulders.
   - Slowly bring your elbows together in front of your, with your arms parallel to the floor.
   - Take your elbows out to the side and back, squeezing your shoulder blades together.
   - Breathe normally.
   - Repeat three more times. Keep your elbows horizontal to the floor throughout.

If you have back or neck problems, exercise caution when doing the following neck and shoulder exercises.

8. **Neck stretch** to relieve headaches:
- Sit upright in your chair, hands resting on your thighs.
- Keeping your back straight, gently lower your chin as close to the chest as you can. The rest of the body remains relaxed. Breathe normally and hold for a few seconds.
- Slowly bring your head up and let it drop back as far as possible, look up and hold for a few seconds.
- Bring your head back to center and tilt it to the right side, keeping your ear aligned with the shoulder. Do not lift your shoulder to meet the ear. Hold for a few seconds.
- Bring your head back to center and repeat on the other side.
- Return your head to the center and slowly turn to look over your right shoulder as far as you can. Align the chin with the shoulder. Hold for a few seconds and return to center.
- Repeat over the left shoulder.
- Complete all the movements three more times.

9. **Neck pendulum** – also good for relieving headaches and migraines.
- From an upright position, drop your chin as close to the chest as you can.
- As you inhale, roll and lift your head to one side, only as far as the shoulder, aligning the chin with the center of the shoulder.
- Exhale and lower your chin back to the center.
- Inhale as you lift and roll it to the other side.
- Repeat from side to side six times.

10. **Shoulder rolls**
- Stand in the Mountain Pose (asana 19) or sit upright in your chair. Arms should be totally relaxed at your side.
- Lift both shoulders up toward your ears.

- Roll them in a circle forward, down, back and up to the ears again.
- Repeat in a forward direction three to five times.
- Reverse direction and repeat in a backward direction three to five times.

11. Shoulder squeeze

- From a standing or sitting position, inhale as you squeeze your shoulders up to your ears. Hold for a couple of seconds and then let your shoulders drop with a big sigh – expelling all the air from your lungs.
- Repeat three to five times.

Do not do the eye exercises if you have a detached retina.

Eye exercises

This series of eye exercises works with all of the muscles around the eye and the optic nerve. These are good for everyone but especially for those with eye problems and those who work in front of a computer screen for long periods of time. If you suffer from myopia, regular practice of the following eye exercise can actually improve your vision.

Eye exercise 1

Sit upright in your chair and visualize a very large clock right in front of you. Keep your head and shoulders still, just work with the eyes. Look as far as you can in each direction.

- Look up at the 12.
- Look at the 9.
- Look down at the 6.
- Look at the 3.
- This is the complete circle: do three rotations.
- Reverse and repeat.

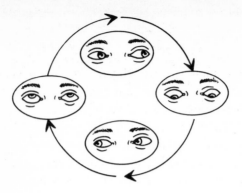

Eye exercise 2

Remain in the same position. Remember to look as far as possible in each direction, without moving your head or shoulders.

- Inhale as you look up at the 12.
- Exhale as you look down at the 6.
- Repeat three times.
- Inhale and look to the 3.
- Exhale and look to the 9.
- Repeat three times.
- Inhale and look up at 1, as far out as you can.
- Exhale and look down at the 7, as close in as you can, almost at the left knee.
- Repeat three times.
- Inhale and look up at the 11, as far out as you can.
- Exhale and look down at the 5, as close in as you can, almost at the left knee.
- Repeat three times.
- Flutter your eyelids for a few seconds to relax the muscles.

Eye exercise 3

This exercise works specifically on the optic nerve as your vision moves from long distance to short distance.

- Hold up your thumb about 30 cm (12 inches) in front of your nose.
- Inhale and look past your thumb into the distance.
- Exhale and look at your thumb.
- Repeat three times.

- Flutter the eyelids for a few seconds.

Eye exercise 4

This exercise works on your peripheral vision.

- With both thumbs up, stretch your arms out directly in front of you with hands together. Your thumbs should be at eye level.
- Maintain a straight back and keep your head still and centered.
- Look at your right thumb and slowly move it sideways. Follow your thumb with your eyes only.
- Stop when you lose sight of your thumb and slowly return your thumb and your eyes to center.
- Repeat three times, then repeat three times with the left thumb.
- Flutter your eyelids for a few seconds.

Eye relaxation exercise

Rub your palms together rapidly for several seconds until you have created a lot of heat in your hands.

- With your fingers closed, place your hands over your eyes – fingertips at the hairline and heels on the cheeks. No light should get through.
- Breathe deeply and hold for a few moments – feel the muscles around your eyes relaxing.
- You should see total black – this means your optic nerve is relaxed. Hold this position for at least five minutes.
- Remove your hands, but keep your eyes closed for a few more seconds.
- Slowly open your eyes.
- If you have degenerating vision do this exercise three times per day for 10 minutes. Otherwise do this exercise after the previous exercises and any time your mind is agitated or your eyes are tired.

Regular practice of the complete breath and the abdominal breath (see Chapter 2) is an important part of every slimming program, as these help melt away superfluous fat from those areas of your body where fat tends to gather.

PROGRAM D: FOR SLIMMING THE BODY

Reduce fat on the sides, waist and thighs

1.   *Triangle* (asana 22)
*   Refer to Chapter 4 for full details.
*   Without pausing, alternate side to side, and repeat a total of nine times on each side.
*   Exhale as you stretch sideways, and inhale as you come up.
*   When complete, gracefully lower the arms to the sides and take three deep breaths.

2.   *Spinal Twist* (asana 12)
*   Refer to chapter 4 for full details.
*   Without pause, slowly repeat nine times on each side.
*   Exhale as you turn toward the side and inhale as you return to center.
*   Do not release your leg until you have completed nine on one side and are ready to switch to the other.
*   When complete, stretch both legs straight ahead and relax. Take three deep breaths.

Reduce fat on hips, buttocks and thighs

1.   *Sitting walk*
*   This exercise requires stamina, but the effects are amazing.
*   Sit on the floor with your legs extended and together.
*   Fold your arms across the chest.
*   Keep your spine straight, thrust forward first with one buttock, hip and leg, then with the other.
*   This is the sitting walk.

- Move forward, thrusting your body forward on each side nine times.
- Move backward nine times on each side.
- Relax; take three deep breaths.
- Repeat the entire exercise, forward and back, two more times.

Reduce fat on abdomen and thighs

1. *Ceiling walk*

- Lie on your back on the floor.
- Inhale and raise your legs until they are perpendicular to the floor. If you have a weak back, you can support your lower spine by placing your hands on your lower back with your fingertips pointing toward the spine. Otherwise leave your arms beside you on the floor.
- Push your heels toward the ceiling.
- Keeping your legs straight, take a long stride, as if you were walking on the ceiling.
- Alternate legs and continue to "walk" while keeping the legs as straight as possible.
- Continue for one to five minutes.
- When you get tired, pretend you are riding a bicycle, first forward for nine circles, then backward for nine circles.
- Bring your legs down and relax with the complete breath for three minutes – you will need it as this exercise also requires a lot of stamina.

Reduce fat from the hips:

1. *Hip circling*

- Stand in the Mountain Pose (asana 19), except have the feet 15 cm (six inches) apart.
- Place your hands on your hips.
- Circle the hips and pelvis slowly in a clockwise direction – nine times.
- Reverse and do nine circles in a counterclockwise direction. (Make the circles as wide as possible.)
- Repeat three more times, in each direction, without pausing.
- Relax and take three deep breaths.

Reduce fat from waist, hips, thighs and buttocks
2. *Leg over*
- Lie on your back with your arms stretched out to the sides.
- Inhale and bring your left knee into your chest then exhale.
- Straighten your left leg up toward the ceiling.
- Bring the left leg over the right leg and lower it toward the floor. (Both shoulders remain on the floor.)
- Without pause, bring the left leg back to the center and lower back to the floor.
- Repeat nine times.
- Repeat with the right leg.
- Relax with the complete breath.

Reduce fat and tone the chin
3. *Chin exercise*
- Sit on the floor or in a chair.
- Slowly bring your bottom jaw forward and up so that the bottom teeth are placed over the upper teeth and you feel a tightening in the chin.
- Relax and repeat nine times without pause.
- Relax with three deep breaths.
- Repeat two more times.
- This is also good for releasing tension in the jaws and reducing teeth grinding during sleep. The Lion (asana 14) is also good for toning the chin.

Reduce flab from arms, chest and bust
4. *Shoulder raise*
- You can do this exercise sitting on the floor or standing up.
- Interlace your fingers behind your back.
- In a slow movement, raise your arms behind your back, as far up as you can without strain.
- Hold for a count of nine.
- Slowly lower your arms and without pausing, repeat nine times, holding each time you raise your arms.
- When complete, separate your hands and rest your arms beside you (if standing) or on your knees (if sitting).
- Take three deep breaths.

Refer to the Shoulder Stand (asana 11) for excellent total weight control. The stimulation of the thyroid gland is an important factor in weight control since this gland is responsible for the metabolic system.

PROGRAM E:
FOR STRENGTHENING THE BACK AND SPINE

There are many exercises that improve the flexibility of the spine, but it is also very important to strengthen the spine. A healthy spine should stretch in four directions, side to side and forward and back. Observe how a cat stretches to appreciate a truly flexible spine. Upon waking, and several times per day, cats automatically bend their spine as far as possible, arching it up and down, to maintain flexibility.

Spine-strengthening exercise

The very best exercise you can do to strengthen the muscles around the spine is the variation of the Squatting Posture (asana 18). Do 12 repetitions and rest as directed. Do this every day and add more repetitions each week until you can complete 25. If you do this every day you will notice the benefits in a very short time. This strengthens muscles of the back and around the kneecap.

Additional spine postures for strength
1. Back Bend (asana 21)
2. Easy Pose (asana 25)
3. Cobra (asana 4) – Repeat without pause 20 times, then rest.
4. Wheelbarrow (asana 10) – repeat without pause 20 times, then rest.

Additional spine postures for flexibility
1. Spread Leg Stretch (asana 2)
2. Back Stretch (asana 3)
3. Plough (asana 5)
4. Dog (asana 6)
5. Boat (asana 9)
6. Bridge (asana 8)

7.   Child Posture (asana 16)
8.   Triangle (asana 22)
9.   Classical Forward Stretch (asana 20)
10. Cat (asana 15)
11. Spinal Twist (asana 12)
12. Warrior (asana 23)

PROGRAM F: TO HELP RELEASE NEGATIVE EMOTIONS

Anger and aggression

Anger is a major cause of ill health. Arguments overwork the adrenal glands and the brain releases too much serotonin, causing an increase in muscle tension and depletion of the immune system. The physiological effects of an argument can last at least three days. Your blood temperature increases and depending on the strength of your anger, it can take three weeks to cool down. It is recommended that you drink a glass of ice water after an argument to help your blood cool down.

During a time of anger, your nerves become weaker, certain blood cells are destroyed and memory power is reduced – observe how forgetful you are after your next argument. Anger is always homemade. Little or no anger means an abundance of happiness.

The recommended asana to combat anger and aggression is the Lion (asana 14). Remember to growl as loud as you can for a better release.

Depression

The Laughasana (asana 13) is the best antidote to depression. Our moods affect our breathing and by changing how we breathe, we can change how we feel. Bad moods or depression act like a broken record in the mind and body, creating a vicious cycle of internal tension and unproductive and negative thoughts, which constrict breathing. Depression is a condition where nothing grows, like stale water. The depressed person has lost sight of what a great gift life is. Becoming thankful for everything there is can lift depression – this is the best medicine for this dark soul condition.

Depression creates acidity in the bloodstream. Become aware of what you eat and try to keep the body alkaline. A good physical workout, not in a gym but cleaning the basement or garage, is highly recommended as a tonic to fight depression. Laugh, laugh, laugh! Stay away from depressing TV shows, movies or books. Buy or rent lots of humorous material that will make you laugh.

Fear

Courage is the antidote to fear, but can sometimes be hard to muster up. We must make a lot of decisions every day and all require courage. These decisions can be as simple as a choice of clothing or food, or as critical as preparing for an important meeting. Sometimes difficulties occur because we cannot make a decision. When we doubt our own abilities, we lose energy.

The Warrior (asana 23) will empower you with a stronger belief system and help you gain more confidence.

Anxiety

The Back Bend (asana 21) can be called an anxiety-releaser. Anxiety is a crippling emotion that prevents you from achieving your highest good or goal. There is a ganglia of nerves near the heart center where anxiety manifests itself. The Back Bend expands the chest to open and stretch this area.

PROGRAM G: FOR PREGNANT WOMEN

During the first trimester of pregnancy it is not recommended for women to do any asanas. During this time, your body is establishing a new hormonal balance that can be negatively affected by the strong effect that yoga exercises can have on your hormonal system. After three months, with your doctor's permission, you can resume a modified yoga exercise routine. Excessive stretching is not recommended at any time during pregnancy due to the increased level of certain hormones that naturally loosen your joints in preparation for childbirth. The rectus abdominal muscle that reaches from the sternum to the pubic bones also loosens during pregnancy and it is not recommended to do any back bends. Also, do not practice meditation during pregnancy as you could injure the fetus with this powerful energy.

Relaxation in the Total Relaxation Posture (asana 1), combined with deep breathing, the alternate nostril breath and affirmations, is highly recommended during pregnancy. This training will help your concentration and ability to relax as you go into labor.

Postures and exercises to prepare for giving birth

1. From Program A

- Lotus stretch
- Dancing star

2. From Program C

- Mountain Pose (asana 19)
- Cat (asana 15)
- Child Posture (asana 16) – with the knees far apart
- Squatting Posture (asana 18) and the variation of the Squatting Posture (but no more than 12 repetitions)

Swimming is also highly recommended as part of your pregnancy exercise routine.

You can improve your health (and the health of the fetus) right away by changing your diet to satvic (pure) food and increasing the amount of time you rest your body and mind.

After you give birth

- Ancient teachings do not recommend any vigorous or strenuous asanas until any bleeding has stopped.
- During delivery all the pores are open, making you susceptible to colds and flu if you are exposed to cold air or cold water during the first four weeks after giving birth.
- Make sure your baby is kept warm immediately after birth.

CHAPTER SIX

Nutrition for yoga and better health

GUIDELINES FOR EATING BEFORE AND AFTER EXERCISE

It is best to practice yoga on a fairly empty stomach so try to practice at least two hours after a large meal or one hour after a light meal. Practicing first thing in the morning is best. Do not drink beverages with caffeine or alcohol before practicing; these stimulate the system and are counterproductive to the goals of yoga.

Drink water that is not too cold to quench your thirst and eat fresh fruit for a quick energy boost. Naturally sweet drinks, fruit juices or a teaspoon of honey are recommended if you are tired after practice.

A good plan for a practice day is to wake early, drink a glass of warm water and empty your bladder and bowels. Then select and practice a yoga program from Chapter 5 that feels good for you. Don't eat anything other than fruit until at least 12 noon. When you sleep at night, your body goes into a state of rest because you do not ingest food for a long period of time. Filling your empty stomach with heavy, hard-to-digest food first thing in the morning shocks the body and requires excessive energy for digestion. Fruit provides your body with a quick source of energy without exacting a lot of energy for digestion.

EVERYDAY DIET CONSIDERATIONS

If those of us in the West treated our bodies with the same care we devote to our automobiles, we could be among the healthiest people in the world. As proud North American car-owners we would never feed our car the equivalent of a coffee and sugar donut for breakfast every morning. The consequences of abusing our cars are often immediately obvious and expensive to repair. Even though cars are replaceable and our bodies are not, most of us are not nearly this diligent with our bodies.

We are fortunate to live in a society with an ample and varied supply of fresh food and clean water, yet we have among the highest rates of cancer and heart disease in the world. When we abuse our bodies with poor food choices, lack of sleep or overconsumption of alcohol and drugs, we do damage that may not surface for many years. Even though we constantly hear and read new research demonstrating the need to improve our diet and lifestyle habits, it can be difficult to make the necessary changes. We are inundated constantly by advertising designed to whet our appetites for the many products we know are bad for us and this can make it very stressful to make sudden major lifestyles changes.

Yoga is about balance and approaching everything we do with moderation, including diet. When you start to practice yoga, start also to educate yourself in some of the yogic principles of diet and lifestyle. Slowly incorporate small changes into your life. Start by making changes to what you eat and drink before and after you practice yoga and pay attention to how you feel.

 Each and every one of us can achieve good health. It involves listening to our bodies. Once we learn this art, many illnesses can be overcome by allowing the body to heal naturally, rather than masking the symptoms with drugs. Each of us has a slightly different constitution – you need to discover which foods suit you best.

As your health and body awareness increase, you should also start to notice how tired or stressed you feel after a fattening fast-food meal and how positive and energized you feel when you eat healthful, fresh food. Noticing these differences is the first step toward making long-term changes in your nutrition and lifestyle choices. You don't have to force major changes all at once – just learn to pay attention to your body, educate yourself and start to make choices on a daily and even hourly basis that leave you feeling positive and stressfree. Start to treat your body as though it were the most valuable, irreplaceable vehicle you will ever own: because it is.

TRADITIONAL YOGA NUTRITION AND PRINCIPLES

Traditional yogins usually follow a strict lacto-vegetarian diet based on ayurvedic principles. (Lacto-vegetarians do not eat animal flesh of any kind, but include milk products in their diet.) Ayurveda, the science of self-knowledge, breaks foods into three basic groups: satvic – pure food; rajasic – stimulating food; and tamasic – impure food.

Satvic food is the purest food and the most suitable for a serious student of yoga. A satvic diet includes organic fresh fruit, vegetables, pure fruit juices, seeds, whole grains, sprouts food, low-fat dairy products, nuts, honey and herb teas. These will nourish the body and purify the mind to promote a peaceful, calm state.

Rajasic food includes very hot, bitter, sour, dry or excessively salty food and includes fish, eggs, chocolate, caffeine and any strong herbs. These stimulating foods destroy the energy equilibrium between the mind and body by stimulating the body and leaving the mind restless and uncontrollable. Eating in a hurry is also considered rajasic.

Tamasic food offers no direct benefit to the body or the mind. This group includes alcohol, meat (this includes all flesh, not just beef), tobacco, overcooked food, fermented foods such as vinegar and stale or overripe substances. Intake of these substances puts substantial strain on the body and reduces our energy and our ability to resist disease. Ancient teachings say tamasic food fills the mind with dark emotions such as anger and greed. Overeating is also considered tamasic.

The teachings of Ayurveda also state that most of your food should be eaten raw to gain the strength-giving vital essence. Cooking food destroys most of its enzymes and vitamins so eating only cooked foods means that you starve your body of the necessary elements it needs for health and ultimately survival.

The basic ayurvedic principles are in complete conflict with our fast-paced Western lifestyle where meals are often picked up and eaten on the way to the next commitment. Again, it would be very stressful on you and your family to attempt an overhaul of your complete lifestyle in a short time. Remember balance and moderation, pay attention to and repeat what promotes positive responses and slowly eliminate those activities that create negative, stressful situations for you and your family.

The rhythmic cycle: from ancient teachings

12 noon – 8 p.m.	food intake and digestion
8 p.m. – 4 a.m.	food assimilation and absorption
4 a.m. – 12 noon	food waste elimination

Breakfast Start the day with a glass of lukewarm water to wash the body internally. Eat only fruit in the morning. Remember this is the time of cleansing and healing for the body.

Lunch Eat porridge in the winter. The rest of the year you can have a salad that includes grated cabbage (to combat breast cancer), raw potatoes (good for the heart), carrots (good for the eyes) and lots of sprouts (full of enzymes). Use organic olive oil or nettle oil combined with lemon juice as a dressing.

Supper Include vegetables, steamed or fried in ghee (clarified butter), organically grown grains, legumes, tofu and all vegetables, especially green leafy vegetables that cleanse the blood.

Milk Milk is a food type, not a drink, so it should be taken separate from meals – half an hour before or after eating. Use milk that is produced using organic regulations.

Drinking Drinking during a meal is not recommended because it dilutes the hydrochloric acid used in the stomach for digestion. Take liquids 15 minutes before or after a meal.

Protein Non-meat sources of protein include nuts, tofu, legumes, algae, beans, tempeh, grains and eggs (in moderation).

VEGETARIANISM

Vegetarianism has been practiced in the East by millions of people for thousands of years. Indian yogins choose to be vegetarians for both health and ethical reasons. In order to reach enlightenment, the ultimate goal, a dedicated yoga student must come to recognize the link between purity of diet and purity of spirit.

From a health perspective, there are many well-documented findings that raise concerns about the long-term damage that meat consumption can cause to our health. Our bodies do not digest meat as quickly or easily as fruit and vegetables. When meat putrefies in our digestive tract, many damaging toxins are released into the body. The intestines of the average meat-eating person become increasingly clogged with putrefactive debris. This debris collects along the wall of the lower intestines, bowel and colon, releasing toxins and blocking its normal function. As blood circulates through the body, it is supposed to absorb nutrients through the intestinal walls to nourish all organs, but this build up of toxic material prevents this natural transfer. This results in the increase of both short-term problems like headaches and confusion, and many longer-term problems and diseases like cancer.

Our greatest source of energy is the sun, and since plants harness and store the sun's energy through photosynthesis, the most direct method to transfer this energy to our body is through ingesting lots of fresh fruit and vegetables. Vegetables and fruit ferment if eaten after food that digests more slowly, so it is imperative to eat fruits, vegetables and other fermenting food first. Eating fruit on an empty stomach is best because it only stays in the stomach for 10 to 20 minutes.

Beyond the health concerns there are the ethical issues associated with killing for food. Animals have nervous systems, they experience pain and can even cry at the loss of a mate or offspring. Current mass-production operations disregard the discomfort, fear or pain thresholds of animals in the methods used to raise, transport and kill them. In a society overflowing in supplies of healthy fruits, vegetables and grains, there is no real necessity to continue to kill animals for food.

The human body shares more characteristics with vegetarian animals than it does with carnivorous animals, indicating that man has chosen to eat meat throughout his evolution more from necessity or convenience than health. Our teeth are designed for chewing grains and our intestines are almost 10 metres long – far too long for digesting meat properly. When we eat meat, it stays in the stomach for four hours and then can stay in the intestines for 72 hours. This process releases damaging toxins into our bodies.

Some additional dietary considerations

- Avoid heavily processed food, such as white bread, white sugar, white rice; artificially sweetened and colored food; heavily sugared drinks such as pop; highly spiced food; and highly salted food (which just about eliminates anything available from the local fast-food franchise).
- Increase your intake of (satvic) fruit and vegetables. Fruit and raw vegetables contain antiscorbutic substances that contain important healing properties.
- Include organic milk and dairy products (including yogurt with live culture and rennet-free cheese) in your daily diet.
- Make half of your daily food intake uncooked food.
- Keep meals simple by having just a few different foods at each meal and include fresh, natural and uncooked foods.
- Eat moderately. (The yogic equation for food intake is to fill half the stomach with food, one-quarter with water and leave one-quarter empty for practicing pranayama.) Regardless of your level of commitment to yoga, it is wise to always stop eating before you are full.
- Always try to eat the locally grown, organic, non-irradiated food that is in season and has not been genetically engineered.
- Chew your food well. This is the first step in the digestive process and it is very important. Saliva, mixed with well-chewed food, creates less strain on the stomach and organs

when processing food. As well as increasing the flavor and enjoyment of the meal, thorough mastication is also a yoga exercise and eating should be performed with your full attention. Many digestive problems are caused when improperly chewed food is ingested – proper breathing during eating is also important.

- Never eat when you are angry or in a hurry.
- Prepare food for yourself and others with love.
- Take a moment to be thankful for your food before each meal. The repetition of this routine will physically trigger the gastric juices to prepare for food.

The availability of foods that are grown and prepared without chemical fertilizers, pesticides, radiation or genetic engineering will only increase through consumer demand. An increase in demand should cause an increase in supply and a corresponding reduction in price. It is in everyone's best interest to encourage farmers and stores to produce and sell foods that promote good general health.

CHAPTER SEVEN

Affirmations

My thoughts today become my reality tomorrow.

An affirmation is a strong, positive statement that expresses the goal you wish to achieve. Affirmations help reverse emotional negativity. When affirmations are repeated several times, a new chain of neurons in the brain is activated, replacing the old, negative thought patterns with positive thought patterns. It takes patience and persistence to fully clear the body of the effects of these negative thought patterns. The blueprint of this negativity is set in your DNA. The first six weeks spent repeating affirmations are very important because this is the length of time it takes for the DNA to replicate itself. As the body begins to clear the blueprint of negativity, the cells release and eliminate the chemistry of fear, anxiety, depression and anger – the emotional reactions attached to this blueprint.

An affirmation must be positive, personal, in the present tense and short. For example, don't say, "I will be decisive," say, "I AM decisive." The truth of the statement is not the point. The point is that by giving your belief system the mental experience of being decisive, you then begin to bring the desired thought into physical manifestation.

Just as indulging in alcohol, drugs and improper diet and lifestyle can weaken our bodies, our minds are susceptible to the mental toxins of fear, anger, envy and impatience. Lasting happiness does not come from having many possessions. True, lasting happiness arises naturally when we become free of the mental and emotional toxins that poison us. The sources of misery are not found outside of us; they are created by us and exist within us. Our own negative emotions agitate the mind.

We create our own experiences by the way we think. The philosopher Henry David Thoreau said, "Many men lead lives of quiet desperation" – the fact is that many women do also. Much of that quiet desperation (or not so quiet) is the result of having to march to the beat of a drummer that is not of our own making. Societal pressure to conform starts in our youth and follows us most of our lives. Many people are willing to pay for their success by sacrificing their health and their relationships to others. It is important to discover, decide and follow only what is truly important to you. We start to change the undesirable pressure of society by first changing its power over us.

Happiness is an individual experience that does not mean the same thing to each person. Ask yourself what it is that you really want. Remember that your thoughts create your reality and the reality around you. If you don't like some area of your life, if there is something you wish to see changed, change your mental approach first. You have freedom of choice and free will. Scientists say that 85,000 to 92,000 thoughts pass through your brain every day. You are responsible for each thought that you think. If you think in a limited or disharmonious manner and dwell on envy, illness and unhappy situations, your attention is on the effect of the problem, rather than the cause. You will continue to reproduce and recreate the same undesirable situations and conditions as long as you proceed in this way. If you think in a creative, healthy, positive and loving way, little by little, you will raise your consciousness to a higher level. You will begin to create a positive reality for yourself and for those around you.

 Think good thoughts, speak good words and read good things. This will give you spiritual strength. What you believe forms your reality. If you cultivate negativity, your reality will be negative. If you cultivate positive thoughts, soon your reality will be positive.

It is easy to think of yourself as a puppet on a string or a slave to the many thoughts and emotions that cross your mind every day. By doing this you give away your power and give up responsibility for your own reality. It is also selfish to expect others to be responsible for your happiness. You are the author of your life – write it well. Most of our behavior and thought patterns are learned when we are very young. Our emotions are also learned responses. If we can learn them, then we can unlearn them. At some point in our lives, we can choose to stop being a slave to the emotions and negativity that have previously controlled our reality. Affirmations are a powerful tool to help us change these long-held patterns of thought and emotion.

Sometimes we find ourselves repeatedly facing the same problems and failures, year after year. It is not bad luck that finds you involved in the same type of bad relationship over and over again. It is your choice. And until you stop and find the courage to examine the problem and learn the proper lessons, you will continue to make the same mistakes. If your life had been "perfect" from the start, you wouldn't have faced a single problem and you wouldn't have learned a single lesson. The challenge to overcome a tough situation is to make it a great opportunity for growth and learning. What you make of your life is entirely up to you and by learning to work on yourself through yoga and affirmations, you can create the positive reality that you desire.

Remember that what you think and wish for another always comes back to you – both positive, loving intentions and negative, harmful intentions. This is a universal law.

Start each day with love and live the day with love. Pay attention to the many thoughts that go through your mind each day. You may be surprised at how many times a day you think negative thoughts about yourself and others. Replace these thoughts with positive affirmations. It takes approximately 15 positive thoughts to erase one negative thought. Always follow the four Cs – I am calm, confident, capable and competent. Choose one to three of the following affirmations and repeat them to yourself several times a day, particularly first thing in the morning, after relaxation and before you go to bed.

- I am abundantly able to succeed in every effort that I truthfully designate.
- I am working every day at my purest intentions for the highest good of all.
- I am calm and balanced in body, mind and spirit.
- I have the inner strength to overcome all obstacles.
- I follow through with what I start.
- I release myself from old habits and addictions.
- I now release my entire past.
- I now let go of all accumulated guilt, fear, anger, resentment, jealousy and disappointment.
- All barriers to my full expression and enjoyment of life are now dissolved.
- The light of peace surrounds me and the power of love protects me.
- Every day I am getting better and better.
- Everything is coming easily and effortlessly toward me.
- I am a radiant being, filled with love and light.
- My life is blossoming in total perfection.
- I have everything here and now.
- I am the master of my life.
- I love and appreciate myself just as I am.
- I take responsibility for creating my reality.
- I give myself permission to let go and let life flow.
- In my life all is well.

CHAPTER EIGHT

Relaxation

Deep relaxation, practiced regularly, strengthens the immune system and produces many other medically valuable changes in the body. People suffering from asthma, for instance, find that relaxation helps widen restricted respiratory passages. Diabetics who relax can reduce the amount of insulin required. Chronic and unbearable pain can be significantly relieved through relaxation. Regular periods of relaxation can also help reduce our susceptibility to viruses, bacteria and disease.

During times of stress, our sympathetic nervous system reacts by secreting hormones that mobilize the body's muscles and organs to face the perceived immediate threat – whatever the threat may be. This is called the fight-or-flight response. This biological response includes shifting blood flow from the limbs to the organs. It causes an increase in blood pressure along with a host of other responses. Everyday worries, anxieties and pressure can also trigger the body's defensive response. Even though there is no immediate danger, the body still physically prepares to fight or flee in response to this type of stress. If the stress is prolonged, the body's repeated preparation to non-existent threat creates wear and tear, leading to dysfunction and debilitation.

Stress is uniquely different from what we normally think of as a disease. It has no biological structure such as germs or viruses; rather it is psychosomatic. Psyche *means mind* – soma *means body.*

Stress comes in different guises. Emotional stress is created by the way we interact with our environment on a day-to-day basis.

Digestive stress is created from poor eating habits and an unhealthy lifestyle. Environmental stress is created through pollution in the air, food and materials that are part of everyday living. Additionally there is stress that stems from our inner habits, including our tendency to focus and blame situations in our life on outside causes. It is this futile attempt to come to grips with these external forces that keeps us from realizing and dealing with the true source of this stress – our own thoughts, feelings and actions.

If something in your life is not working, you need to look at your own belief system and thought processes. You are the true creator of all the situations of your life – if you can create stress, you can dismantle it. A key factor is your ability to take responsibility for your own life. Through certain mental disciplines, you can bring about significant changes in the bodily functions associated with stress.

Modern society has eliminated many of the traditional methods of evoking the body's true relaxation response, such as prayer, chanting and meditation. Yet, in our ever-changing, fast-paced world we need real relaxation more than ever. Rather than taking a coffee break, try taking a total relaxation break. Do not confuse your body's response to this kind of relaxation with ordinary relaxing activities like catnaps, gardening, watching TV, and so on these activities do not invoke the same physiological changes.

True relaxation can be achieved on three levels: the physical body; the nervous system; and the mind. Relaxation and concentration are interdependent.

Do not worry about whether you are successful in achieving a deep level of relaxation. Adopt a passive "let it go" attitude and permit relaxation to occur at its own pace. If a distracting thought enters your mind – let it go. If a happy thought enters – follow it. After some practice you will find a lot of the accumulated cobwebs in your mind disappear and a new perspective on problems will emerge.

BASIC RELAXATION TECHNIQUE

Lie down in the Total Relaxation Posture. Close your eyes and become aware of your breathing, feeling the belly rise and fall with each breath. Inhale and exhale through the nose. As you exhale, feel yourself letting go of tension, worries and anxieties. As you inhale feel the peace and stillness fill you.

 If a troubling issue continues to interrupt your relaxation process, visualize yourself placing it on a shelf. Give yourself permission to set it aside for a short time and say to yourself, "I will deal with this issue later." Just as you plan your work and set some projects aside to be worked on at another time, set your worries aside and give yourself permission to deal with them at a later time. This approach to worries frees your mind to relax.

TENSION / RELAXATION EXERCISE

While in the Total Relaxation Posture, travel mentally through your body starting with the feet and toes. Tighten your feet, work up through the ankles, calves, knees, thighs, hips, lower back, abdomen, stomach, chest, upper back, shoulders, arms, wrists, hands and fingers, and tighten each area, finally clenching the fists. Without releasing the tension in your body, lift your legs, head, upper body and arms a few inches off the floor, feeling the tension in your entire body. As you lift, inhale – hold the breath for as long as if feels comfortable. Be aware of the tension throughout your body.

When you can no longer hold your breath, exhale and allow your body to fall back to the floor naturally. Relax. Take three deep complete breaths. Now mentally travel through the body in the same order, but this time focus on relaxation. With each exhalation, give yourself permission to "let go" more and more. Scan your body for tension and if you still find any, breathe into it and exhale it out through the legs and the soles of your feet. Visualize it disappearing into the earth. There is no need to hold on to anything. Allow your self to be carried by mother earth.

Observe your emotions. If they seem negative or if they seem to obscure the truth, let love and kindness melt them away. Feel the light of the sun shine in your heart. Feel your heart opening, expanding and slowing down. Allow this light to penetrate each cell of your entire being. Feel as though you are basking in the light. Visualize yourself in perfect health. Allow any healing that needs to take place to happen "now."

Choose any scenario where you feel peaceful, safe and calm and visualize this during relaxation. This could include a beach, mountain, forest, waterfall or moonlit sky. Practice in the morning for 10 minutes and in the evening for 15 minutes. The point here is to train yourself to become mindful. If you fall asleep – this may happen in the beginning – you will not reap the physiological benefits of the relaxation response.

CHAPTER NINE

Meditation

Even though we are drowning in information, many of us still thirst for greater internal knowledge and wisdom. Meditation opens you to the existence of this knowledge.

Scientists who have studied the effects of meditation have found that when in the meditative state, the two hemispheres of the brain, which normally generate brain waves of different frequencies, actually synchronize. This synchronization leads to a deeper awareness and intense mental clarity. The effects of meditation include reduced heart rate and blood pressure, improved function of the gastrointestinal tract, relaxation of muscles and an increase in the amount of oxygen and blood flowing to the brain.

The science of meditation was developed systematically in ancient India during the Upanishad period, between 800 and 1200 BC. Indian monks established a school of meditation in the third or fourth century AD and the earliest known meditation school in China dates from 525 AD. Later, teachers travelled to Japan – the word *Zen* is derived from the Sanskrit word *dhyana*, meaning meditation.

The benefits of meditation are twofold: first there are the physical benefits that stem from better stress management, improved posture and increased breath control. But along with the physical changes, those who meditate regularly soon become intensely familiar with the depths of their own consciousness and their true place in the universe. Even if you are not religious at all, meditation will bring you a new and refreshing perspective on life.

As general interest in yoga and other Eastern philosophies has increased in the West, many have realized that we are suffering from spiritual poverty. Even those who have gained enormous material success in life come to realize these accomplishments do not guarantee happiness and contentment. The direction of Western civilization has always been more focused on outward achievement – producing, building, dissecting and destroying and this greed for material possessions often produces a ruthless competitiveness. If all our energy is focused on having more, we can never find fulfilment, for no matter what is achieved, more will always be required. The ever-unfulfilled desires and expectations, coupled with overcompetitiveness, usually create feelings of anger, eventually leading to destructive behavior in ourselves, our families and in society.

The vision of Western culture has always been external – searching for meaning outside of human consciousness and the need to conquer nature. In contrast, Eastern spiritual aspirants look within, learning to understand and live in harmony with nature rather than attempting to conquer it. They recognize themselves as part of the whole, a co-creator with the Creator.

Meditation is the tool we use to detoxify the mind. When we open the mind and just learn to observe our thoughts, we can begin to see the source of our difficulties. Diffused power is noise, and concentrated power is stillness. Self-knowledge is the greatest knowledge in the universe. Meditation is a powerful way to learn to access this knowledge, but first we have to train the mind through concentration.

Concentration develops one-pointedness and tranquility. By focusing the mind on one object, like a candle or image of a deity during meditation, you develop the ability to focus on a single object or thought. When you are in meditation, first concentrate on the technique, object or form you have chosen, then pass into contemplation and finally enter meditation. From concentration you must cross the field of contemplation to enter meditation. Be patient and persistent; it is natural for our minds to wander.

One of the consequences of living an achievement-oriented life is that it causes us to become too attached to the material world. These attachments lead to suffering because what we cling to, we must inevitably lose. Everything is transient in this life: your house, car, clothes, job, even your relationships. But those treasures of your inner life – like love, forgiveness and kindness – are of lasting value and transportable to every situation. Meditation reveals your inner self to you, which is your true being, the Atman – the Sanskrit word for Godhead. It also teaches you that life is a gift to be appreciated and loved. It is through these lessons that wisdom and true knowledge is revealed to you.

Through the practice of meditation you can become more aware of your attachments and stop wasting energy by clinging to transient objects. You will also become more conscious of directing the flow of your thoughts, and learn to free yourself from the conditioned responses that keep you on an emotional roller coaster, feeling like and seeing yourself as a victim. Meditation transcends this cycle of cause and effect, broadens and opens our consciousness, leading finally to internal freedom. To achieve true happiness, we must learn to live life in the present, release the past with love and stop worrying about the future.

The past is history, the future is a mystery, and the present is a gift.

When we look deep inside ourselves, we learn how we have created our own suffering. It is from this understanding that we can free ourselves, leading us into stillness and happiness, which is peace. When you have released yourself from your attachments, wisdom arises, bringing forth equanimity, loving, kindness and compassion. When the mind is completely balanced, tranquil and keenly alert, you will experience yourself as a co-creator in this universe and reach nirvana – a state of total bliss.

Meditation is a growth process. It is acquired slowly and haltingly and then only where there is a persistent search, motivated by disciplined desire. It is attuning our mental and physical bodies to their spiritual source, seeking to know our relationship with God, and becoming one with the Godhead. Just as we do not see the stars in the daylight, we may never experience the essence of meditation in the daylight of ordinary activity with all its complexities.

In *How to Know God*, Patanjali says, "The mind turns inward seeking always the cause behind the cause until the innermost reality is reached. Separation ceases to exist. One becomes the Godhead. One returns to the source."

Although there are many ways to reach Atman, one must remember that eventually we must let go of all techniques, dogmas and mantras. We must always focus on the end result, the Creator of the universe.

HOW TO MEDITATE

Choose a special location that you can always use for meditation. This will be a place you can honor and where you won't be disturbed – it can even be in the same area where you practice yoga. Select a time of day that you can reserve for meditation. Treat this time like any other appointment – schedule it as a special item among your daily activities. You are making and keeping an appointment with yourself. It is best to do this work on a daily basis, but a few times a week is also good. The process of maintaining this appointment at a specific time helps your mind become accustomed and prepared to entering the meditative state.

The length of meditation will vary according to your needs and stamina. Initially 10 to 15 minutes will be sufficient for your meditation, and it can be extended to 30 minutes as you become more comfortable.

You can sit in the Easy Posture – this posture represents peace – or you can sit in a chair. If you choose to sit in a chair, do not lean back; sit closer to the edge of the chair, with your feet slightly apart and firmly placed on the floor. Regardless of whether you sit on the floor or on a chair, it is most important to maintain a straight spine throughout the meditation. Do not lie on the floor – it is necessary to be sitting upright in order to get the energy moving through the spine.

It can be useful to start with an object to focus on. Pictures of your deity, a mandala or a candle are all effective objects for meditation. The flame of a candle is a powerful image for meditative reflection because a thousand people can take the flame of one candle to light their own without diminishing the flame of the original.

When you are comfortably seated and sure you will not be disturbed, look at your chosen object for a few minutes with soft eyes. Then close your eyes and visualize the object firmly in your mind. Make sure your spine is straight without causing tension in the shoulders and neck.

On each hand, touch the thumb to the index finger (representing the symbol of knowledge and wisdom) and rest the back of each hand on the corresponding thigh. Place the tip of your tongue gently behind the teeth where the palate starts; this joins the yin and yang channels.

If you find your spine starts to slouch during meditation, slowly and gently correct it each time you become aware of it. It takes time to strengthen the spine, but you will be successful if you keep meditating.

Countless thoughts will pass through your mind. Notice each one without attachment and learn to be an observer of your thoughts. If you get caught up in these thoughts, it will create tension in the body. Each time you find you are being distracted by a thought, gently bring your awareness back to your chosen object.

When you become physically uncomfortable, release yourself slowly and rest for 10 to 15 minutes. Do not lie down and do not talk during this rest period.

Meditate on a word

If it helps, you can meditate on a word like "peace" or "love." Through meditation on "peace," you will be guided by peaceful thoughts and a peaceful nature through all events in your life. If you meditate on "love," feel the great love that exists within you, in the world and that was used to create this beautiful world. Open your mind and heart to this love, sense it and become it.

Sit in the light of true self healing.
Sit in the realization of your true nature.
Experience the truth beyond mind and matter.

CHAKRAS AND CHAKRA MEDITATION

The chakras are subtle, concentrated energy centers within the body. We have SEVEN major chakras running parallel to the physical body, starting from the base of the spine to the top of the head. Each represents a different level of consciousness. The first THREE lower centers are concerned mainly with our physical existence on earth, while the THREE higher chakras correspond to our spiritual self.

The word *chakra* is a Sanskrit term meaning wheel. The chakras are described as whirling funnels of energy and when balanced, the energy in each whirl around in a clockwise direction. Meditating on the chakras helps open and balance each of these centers. These centers also nourish all organs with their energy. They are described below.

First chakra: Muladhara, the root chakra

- located at the base of the spine in the area of the coccyx
- associated color – red
- associated element – earth, representing lethargy
- connects us to our deepest physical nature and contains our will to live
- recognizing the unfolding of the divine potential and rising above the confinement from fear of death

Second chakra: Svadhisthana, the procreative chakra

- located at the sacrum
- associated color – orange
- associated element – water
- connects to the reproductive organs
- all senses connected to this center
- the center of evolving consciousness: respecting the wisdom of the body and learning how to move the energy up instead of losing it down and outward

Third chakra: Manipura, connected to the solar plexus

- located just above the navel
- associated color – yellow
- associated element – fire, relating to the digestive system
- functions in alignment with higher consciousness
- becoming aware that there is more to life than survival and pleasure
- the center for self-discovery – letting go of the ego through the medium of love
- learning to discipline the senses, returning to the unity of consciousness

Fourth chakra: Anahata, connected to the heart center

- located between the breasts, just above the diaphragm
- associated color – emerald green
- associated element – air
- the first center of a higher state of consciousness, realized when we let go of all addictions and attachments
- freedom from confinement, establishing trust within – not through achievement but through discovering who we are
- embracing all conditions in this life with love
- exploring our divine potential

Fifth chakra – Vissudha, connected to the throat center

- located in the area of the throat
- associated color – blue
- associated element – akasa (which relates to things ethereal)
- the center where a higher state of consciousness unfolds (it is not what we have learned, it is what we are; taking responsibility for yourself and becoming totally self-sufficient)
- no longer propelled by karma; free from all struggles

- becoming aware of eternity and living in perfect balance and harmony

Sixth chakra: Ajna, connected to the third eye

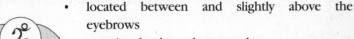

- located between and slightly above the eyebrows
- associated color – deep purple
- the center of polarity of the male and female principles; functioning effectively in mind and body
- the wisdom and guidance center; where the emergence of the inner guru takes place
- one no longer identifies with the body, mind or emotions but experiences a constant state of bliss
- receiving direct guidance from the Inner Source
- transformation from duality toward unity and integration occurs at this level of consciousness

Seventh chakra: Sahasrara, connected to the crown center

- located at the top of the head
- associated color – violet
- represented by the thousand-petal lotus flower
- cosmic energy is stored in this center (it is the main switch that allows the thousand rays of life current to maintain the thousand functions of the body)
- one remains established in one's Source. One is eternally present in all things and forms. There are no boundaries.

The heart chakra is at the center of the seven, and is considered the bridge between the lower and the higher chakras. Our lower three chakras are often blocked or damaged for many reasons including growing up in an abusive or dysfunctional environment. It is imperative to give these lower chakras your attention first. Usually they require a lot of healing before you can move up to work with the higher chakras. It is important to keep in mind that there is nothing negative about an energy blockage; it is simply a lesson that needs to be learned. When all the chakras are in perfect balance and harmony, the result is perfect health in body, mind and spirit. This journey can only be attained by loving and nourishing ourselves.

In the base of your spine you have a tiny little nerve coiled around three times; it is the thickness of a thin hair. Ancient teachings call this the sleeping serpent. When you meditate, pray or chant, this sleeping serpent starts to raise its head and touch the spinal column, releasing a tremendous amount of energy. This is called kundalini energy or serpent power. The chakras represent the stages of the ascent of this power. Nirvana or bliss consciousness is experienced when the kundalini energy travels up through the sushumna channel, through each chakra until it reaches the crown chakra.

When you first start meditating, it is important to focus on the first chakra until you can feel a sensation like tingling or warmth. This may take a few weeks or a month. After you feel a sensation in the first chakra you are ready to begin working on the second chakra, applying the same technique as for the first, then move to the third and so on to the seventh chakra. Finally you will be able to work through every chakra each time you meditate. If you are good at visualization, visualize the colors associated with each chakra, in each energy center. If that is not easy for you, simply focus on what each chakra represents.

Chakra meditation

Combine this with the meditation practice described above. First familiarize yourself with the following meditation and with the location and associated aspects of each chakra. The basic premise is to connect to the earth's energy through the first chakra and slowly work your way up, opening and experiencing each chakra as you go.

Let your posture be without strain and tension.
Breathe deeply into the core of your being.
Release all tension and holding.
Relax your jaw and facial muscles.
Relax your palms and open them.
All tensions are now resolved.
Allow your body to open and receive the universal energy.

Visualize the "white light" all around you.

Visualize a red glowing energy in your coccyx (first chakra).

Allow the energy to rise up into your sacrum (second chakra). See it as a warm orange, deeply nurturing and satisfying.

Allow the energy to rise up into your solar plexus (third chakra). See it as radiant sunshine – yellow – see and feel the yellow light streaming into your solar plexus, dissolving all anxieties and worries.

Allow the energy to rise up into your chest (fourth chakra) in a beautiful emerald green – feel your heart open. Open yourself to the universe to receive the highest energy form this moment has to offer.

Allow the energy to rise to your throat (fifth chakra) in a rich blue – feel the stillness, calmness and peacefulness. Release all your connections; it is safe to let go – this is the center where all dualities and thought forms come together. Feel the power and the truth that you are.

Allow the energy to rise up to the third eye – the space between your eyes (sixth chakra). See it as a rich royal purple. Know and understand the stillness and the divinity within you.

Totally attune yourself to the life force coming from the base of your spine, all the way up to the crown of the head (seventh chakra). Visualize a beautiful violet and a thousand-petal lotus flower. Place your soul in communion with the divine; allow yourself to receive wisdom – that which has no beginning and no end. Every cell is filled with the full spectrum and the highest energy available at this moment.

Now allow all the energies to merge into a white shimmering diamond light.

Allow yourself to be and experience this life force.

Shanti means peace on the physical, emotional and spiritual level. The best investment you can make is to stay healthy. You only reap what you sow, so take great care in what you eat and lead a regular life. Remember your body is a moving temple. Shanti is internal peace connected to your life force. Your life force can only flow correctly when you are peaceful. Shanti creates a total balance between yin and yang and is a force that protects you from all sickness. Shanti is a state where the body, soul and spirit are in total harmony. It is not the viruses and bacteria that bring about our illnesses, or the medicine that makes us healthy – it is the mind that creates your state of being and it is inner peace that creates and sustains perfect health. What you think now, you will become tomorrow.